FITNESS
OVER 40

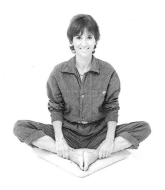

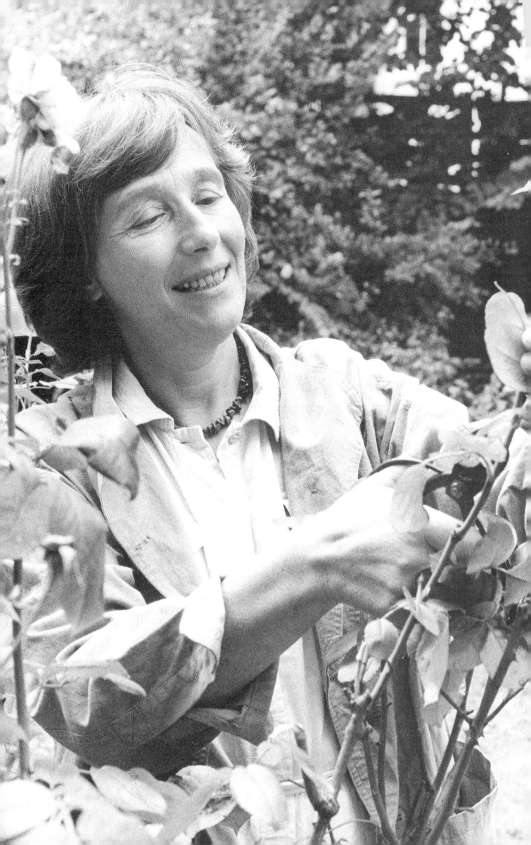

FITNESS OVER 40

A woman's guide to mid-life health,
emotional wellbeing and exercise

JANE LAGESSE
&
HELGE RUBINSTEIN

Photographs by Anthea Sieveking

THE BODLEY HEAD
LONDON

To Barbara Dale,
with love and thanks
J.L.

For my mother and
my daughter
H.R.

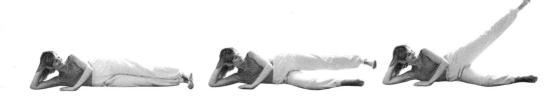

Fitness over 40: A woman's guide to
mid-life health, emotional wellbeing and exercise
was conceived and produced
by Frances Lincoln Limited
Apollo Works, 5 Charlton Kings Road, London NW5 2SB

First published in Great Britain by
The Bodley Head 30 Bedford Square, London WC1B 3RP

British Library Cataloguing in Publication Data
Lagesse, Jane
Fitness over forty.
1. Middle age – Health and hygiene
I. Title II. Rubinstein, Helge
613'.0434   RA777.5

ISBN 0 370 30706 2 hardback
      0 370 30707 0 paperback

CONTENTS

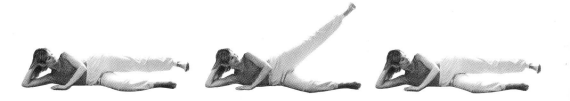

INTRODUCTION

Every generation, at least since the Victorian age, has probably considered itself to be living through an era of transition. Women now in their 40s and 50s are no exception: the last twenty years have been an extraordinary period of accelerated change in how we are seen and how we see ourselves.

The Women's Movement, whether we have been personally active in it or no, has affected us all, and one of its greatest benefits has been that, for the most part, women can now be women, and no longer need to strive to be 'girls'.

Women are coming into their own, and we are the beneficiaries of the new wave of self-awareness and self-confidence. At the same time, while most of the men with whom we have grown up have welcomed the feminist revolution, they are also often mature enough not to have lost confidence in their role as men.

Though we may have been raised in a climate where girls still came second-best to boys, and may lack the determined confidence that our daughters have, ours is probably the first generation of mature women who can dare to be feminine yet confident, and who do not have to apologise either for being women or for our maturity.

Reaching a happy plateau

Women now in their early 50s were recently described as having 'developed a kind of easy, energetic flamboyance and magnetism' and 'a delighted confidence at having left behind at last their repressed early youth, followed by their wild revolutionary late youth. They have "arrived" on a happy plateau . . .'

'A happy plateau' is a much more positive term than 'middle-aged', which conjures up pictures of spare tyres, balding heads and great wastes of disappointed hopes or resigned boredom. Gertrude Stein called her middle years her 'late youth', while Victor Hugo described the 40s as 'the old age of youth' and the 50s as 'the youth

This may be the time to take up a new career or just to develop and enjoy special skills.

6

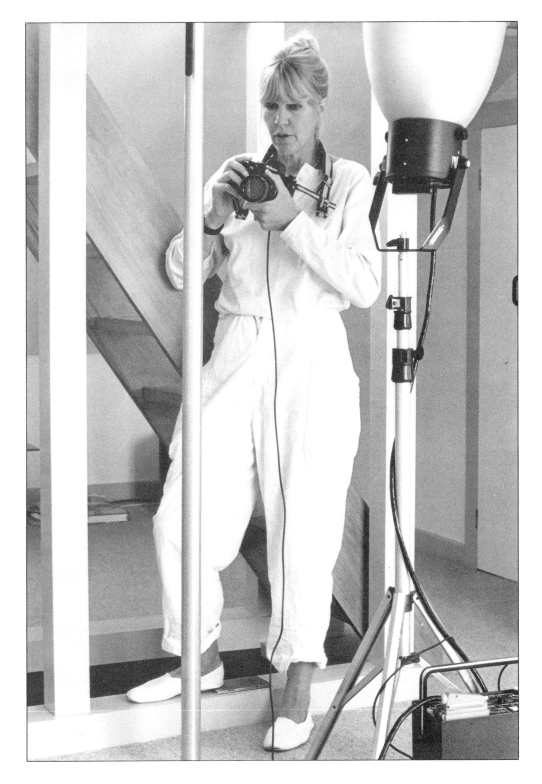

of old age'. Whichever euphemism we may use, we have to come to terms, sooner or later, with the fact of our aging.

But acceptance can be active and positive: very different from passive resignation. The term 'mid-life crisis' may lurk at the back of all our minds, but though 'crisis' has taken on a largely negative tint, we should remember that it comes from the Greek word for decision – an excellent watch-word for this time in our lives. There are a lot of decisions we can make.

At 40 a woman is only half-way through her natural adult lifespan and can face the future with mental and physical energy and zest.

We can decide that along with the losses, there are also gains, many of them considerable (which of us indeed would willingly live again through our adolescence and early youth?). Most of us have a

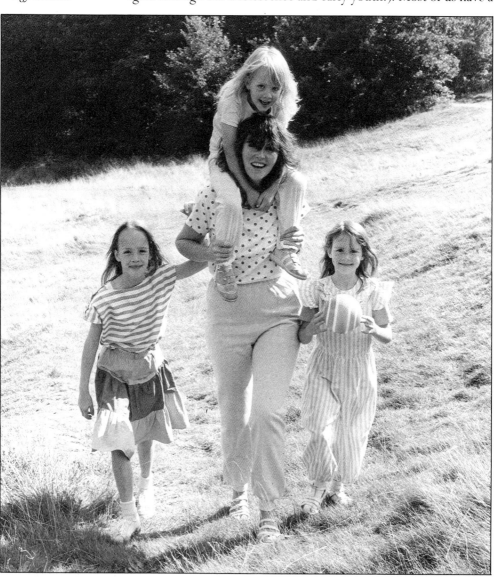

much clearer idea of who and what we are. We no longer need to live out the picture that others have of us, nor focus our lives on meeting other people's needs. We can finally now, and often for the first time, decide to recognize our strengths as well as our weaknesses, acknowledge our own tastes and interests, meet our own needs and take charge of our own lives. It can be liberating, as well as a little scary, to make a realistic assessment of ourselves, and not to see ourselves through the eyes of others and of their wishes, needs and demands on us.

The half-way mark

Middle-age does indeed mean that we are half-way through our natural adult life-span. We are at the middle, not at the end, and there is an urgency for many of us to use the coming years well, to make them as productive and as enjoyable as we can.

This can take many forms. Some women become physically or mentally adventurous, pitting their physical strength and endurance, or their mental energies and skills, against new challenges. For others the challenge may lie in being less busy, in cultivating inner strengths, quiet skills and closer relationships. Nor are these two ways mutually exclusive.

Whichever direction our lives take, they are ours, and we must take responsibility for them. Moreover the stark facts are that since there are more of us than ever before (everyone now in their 40s is part of the post-war baby-boom, and on the whole women live longer than men) the vast majority of us will ultimately have to take care of ourselves.

Acceptance and understanding

So it behoves us now to take care of our bodies as well as our minds. However much we may once have refused to believe that we would ever move towards old age, we must now accept that relentless process; the only alternative to acceptance is rage, frustration and despair.

In order to accept, we have to understand. In order to take care of our mental and physical well-being and balance — and the physical, mental and emotional are closely allied and interdependent — we have to understand what is happening to our bodies and in our lives, and to learn how we can best help ourselves to be as fit and healthy as possible. Eating a sensible diet and taking regular exercise enable us to meet the new challenges. Many older women taking up exercise for the first time are amazed by how much they can achieve.

Just as knowledge and training for childbirth has been helping generations of women to accept and welcome the process of birth, instead of increasing the pain by fighting it, so a similar knowledge and understanding of the physiological changes and emotional fluctuations of the menopause and the middle years should help us not only to accept this stage in our lives too, but also to make the most of our mental and physical strengths, and to increase our well-being. We hope that this book will help women to do so.

THE CHALLENGE OF PHYSICAL CHANGE

Aging is as natural and as inevitable as being born and growing up, yet, while we celebrate births and birthdays in childhood and youth, the older we get, the more women especially seem to dread growing older still. This is sad, since maturity has many compensations, such as more free time (particularly once children have left home), the confidence that experience of life brings to relationships both new and old, and, for women, release from the domination of the menstrual cycle once the menopause is complete.

Yet the menopause has for generations been approached by women with muted fear. Many of us can probably remember our own mothers talking as mysteriously about their 'time of life' as they had once talked about the 'time of the month', alluding darkly to 'the change' and having hushed conversations with their friends. Often this was at a time that was difficult for us too, struggling with the doubts and conflicts of adolescence, and here were our mothers suddenly inexplicably emotional, volatile or depressed. No wonder the menopause tends to appear as a threatening cloud looming on the horizon as we enter our fifth decade.

An end and a beginning

Women have become used to experiencing the major landmarks of life in their bodies much more markedly, dramatically even, than men do. The onset of menstruation, pregnancy and childbirth – these are all turning-points in our lives, with far-reaching repercussions on all our relationships and activities, and especially also on how we think of ourselves. They all centre on the womb, which can feel at these times like the most essential part of the self. It is not surprising therefore when it comes to the menopause and the end of the womb's active life that women are anxious and confused.

It *is* a time of change, and the older we are, the harder it becomes to welcome change. Change implies the end of one era, with the loss of the familiar, and the beginning of another, which is unknown.

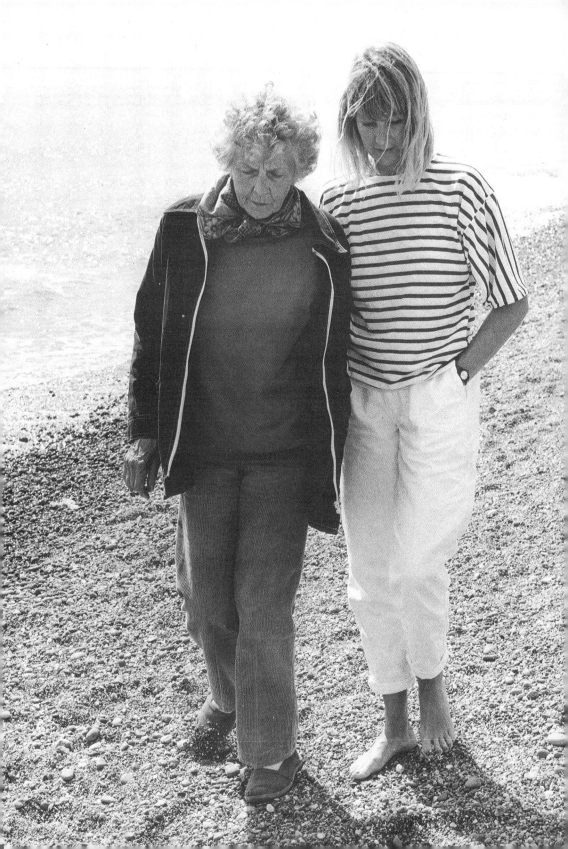

For many women, the menopause seems only to mean loss, whereas there is much to be gained as well, but first there is a necessary transition period to be gone through, both physically and mentally.

Although this chapter and the next will deal mostly with the physical changes of middle life, it is impossible to separate the physical from the emotional, for the two are always inextricably linked (see pages 35 and 67). The more positive the approach to the menopause, the better will be the experience of it, and the most important service we can do ourselves is to demythologize it. The anticipation is often worse than what is actually experienced, probably because of the myths younger women hear associated with it and the attitudes of a youth-orientated society to 'older' women. As one woman said, 'I was pleasantly surprised that the symptoms were really little more than exaggerated feelings of heat. It was just rather unnerving because it was unpredictable.' The menopause will be every woman's reality in time, and the best way to approach it is to understand as fully as possible what is actually taking place in our bodies during this period. There was a world-wide bestseller in the 1920s called *Love* (which meant Sex) *Without Fear*. Perhaps this chapter should be called 'Menopause Without Fear'.

What is the menopause?

The menopause (from the Greek words for month and ending) is, strictly speaking, the moment when a woman's menstrual periods cease. However it has come to be used commonly for the time during which a woman comes to the end of that part of her life when she is able to conceive and bear a child, a time which is more correctly known as the 'climacteric'. Though the two are linked, they are not exactly the same: the menopause is the final punctuation mark when a woman menstruates for the last time; the climacteric describes the span of years during which the various changes take place in her body that lead to the decline and end of the reproductive process, and during which the body adjusts to these changes and prepares for the next, non-reproductive, phase of life.

Ending the reproductive process

Every woman is born with about half a million egg cells already stored in the ovaries. The number diminishes over the years, but during her reproductive period she may produce between three and four hundred ova: nature is prodigal in the cause of survival. Each month an egg ripens in response to the follicle-stimulating hormone (FSH for short) and is released into the uterus. The womb prepares to receive the egg by a thickening of its lining (the endometrium), but if the egg is not fertilized and so does not implant itself in the wall of the womb, this spongy tissue is broken down and sloughed off as part of the menstrual flow. Meanwhile the ovum, as it ripens, produces oestrogen, and after it has travelled into the uterus the follicle from which it has been released produces progesterone and also some oestrogen.

As a woman grows older, the supply of eggs gradually diminishes and the ovaries become less responsive to FSH. The monthly periods become irregular and gradually cease altogether. But this does not mean that the body stops producing these sex hormones. Both oestrogen and progesterone continue to be manufactured, though in lesser quantity than before, and are released into the bloodstream by the other endocrine (hormone-producing) glands, notably the adrenals. There is a period of imbalance while the body adjusts to this new pattern: not only the ovaries and the endocrine glands, but also the womb, the vagina and the breasts are affected, and so is the nervous system. Hormones act as chemical messengers between the various organs and the brain so that even thoughts and emotions are sensitive to the functioning of the glands, and as their hormone production fluctuates, so may a woman's moods (more of this in the next chapter). Eventually the hormonal system reaches a new equilibrium, though at a lower level than before the onset of the menopause: the climacteric is over, and the next phase of life has begun.

When does it start?

Most women start the menopause in their mid to late 40s, and most have completed the process by their early to mid 50s, but there are considerable variations at both ends, and especially in the age of the onset of the menopause. It used to be thought that women who started to menstruate early would stop later (that they were endowed with a greater initial stock of ova) but there is no real evidence for this; what does seem to be the case is that there is a hereditary link, and that those whose mothers had a late menopause may expect to have the same. There are no hard and fast rules, but it is statistically true that just as the menarche (onset of periods) begins earlier these days, so, with better nutrition, there is a tendency in the West towards a later onset of the menopause.

How it begins: irregular periods

The first sign that the menopause has begun is usually that the periods become irregular. There is no one set pattern for this; the variations within what is normal are as great as are the variations in how women experience their monthly periods before the menopause begins.

Probably the most common pattern is for the menstrual flow to become progressively lighter, sometimes with the occasional heavy period in between, to last for fewer days and for the intervals between periods to lengthen until eventually they tail off completely. Some women find that their periods alternate between being very heavy and very light, others that at first they miss out the occasional period, then this happens increasingly until they have stopped altogether. A very few women simply continue to have normal periods until one day they stop and never start again.

Heavy bleeding

Sometimes a woman suffers from exceptionally heavy or

prolonged bleeding. If this happens just once or twice, it is probably due to the temporary imbalance of the hormones, which occasionally stimulate an excessive development of the endometrium. This then results in heavy menstrual bleeding or 'flooding'; in other words, though the bleeding is much heavier than usual, it can still more or less be contained in the usual way with tampons or sanitary towels. If this happens quite frequently, you should consult your doctor, even though there is likely to be little cause for alarm. He may suggest temporary hormone treatment (see page 16), or a check for anaemia, which can be treated with iron supplements.

Heavy bleeding can also be caused by fibroids in the uterus. These small non-malignant growths in the uterine wall are a development of excess muscle and tissue and are extremely common: in fact it has been estimated that 1 in 5 (some say 1 in 3) women over the age of 40 has these harmless growths. Fibroids are easy for the doctor to discover by manual examination in the surgery, and they can if necessary be removed (see p.28). However, if they do not cause too much discomfort, the doctor may decide to wait until the menopause is completed, as most fibroids will shrink during this period and then cause no further problems.

You should always consult your doctor if the bleeding is really heavy or continues without a break. It is especially important to seek medical help *instantly* if there is haemorrhaging – that is, if it is impossible to contain the flow of blood – or if there are clots in the blood. You should also see your doctor if you have bleeding or spotting between periods or after intercourse. These symptoms are not necessarily alarming, but they should always be medically checked, at any age.

If your periods come to a sudden stop, you should also check with your doctor. Don't assume that this is the beginning of the menopause, especially if you are in your early or mid 40s. Some illnesses can interrupt the pattern of menstruation, and so can stress or shock, bereavement or other major life changes. And don't rule out the possibility that you could be pregnant!

Continuing contraception

When a woman's periods become irregular at this stage, it probably means that ovulation has also become sporadic, but it is possible during this time for her to menstruate without actually ovulating. The ovarian follicles may no longer release an ovum each month, but the womb continues to respond to the hormonal messages and to prepare itself for an ovum as before. The lining thickens and is then sloughed off just as though an unfertilized egg is being shed in the normal course of menstruation. Just occasionally the opposite can also happen and a woman may ovulate without menstruating.

This unpredictable pattern of menstruation and ovulation during the menopause means that it is important to continue with contraception if you don't want to risk having a 'menopause mistake' baby. The younger you are the more likely it is that you are still ovulating, so it is even more important to take precautions against becoming pregnant, even if your periods seem to have stopped.

Choosing the best method

Taking the contraceptive pill becomes less safe as you get older. The risk of blood clotting as a result of taking the pill increases, and on the whole women over the age of 40 should no longer be on the pill. Much better to use a diaphragm, or for your partner to use a condom. The IUD (intra-uterine device) suits some women, but there is a risk of infection, and you should have it checked very regularly.

Couples who are in a stable relationship and who are certain that they will not want more children often choose sterilization as the safest method of all. Women may be sterilized by having their fallopian tubes tied or cauterized, an effective method which involves only minor surgery and little risk. More widely practised in America than in England, this is unlikely to be the method of choice at this stage in a woman's life, and it is simpler, and even safer, for the man to have a vasectomy. This can be done in the doctor's surgery, takes less than half an hour to do and carries virtually no risk of after-effects, either physical or psychological. However, neither of these procedures are reliably reversible and neither should be embarked on without careful thought and consultation.

Whichever method of contraception you choose, unless you are sterilized, be sure the menopause is really completed before you stop using it. As a general rule of thumb, if you are under 50, you should continue with contraception for two years after your last period; over 50 twelve months is probably sufficient, although some doctors prefer to recommend that you continue for two years after the last period, whatever your age.

Hot flushes

While the irregularity and gradual or abrupt cessation of menstrual periods are the main and most obvious manifestations of the climacteric, there are also a number of other symptoms, of which the hot flush is certainly the most notorious.

The first thing to say about hot flushes and night sweats is that, although they can be a great nuisance, they are absolutely harmless. No one yet knows precisely what causes them, but they are almost certainly connected with the hormonal changes that are taking place at this time. The fluctuating level of oestrogen in the bloodstream gives erratic messages to the hypothalamus, which acts as the internal body thermostat, thus triggering off the body's heating and cooling mechanisms, often at wildly inappropriate moments.

Almost all women will experience these flushes during the menopause to a greater or lesser degree. They usually begin after the periods have become irregular or diminished, and continue for a year or so; sometimes, though rarely, for several years after the periods have stopped. Some women only have them occasionally, others can have bouts of three or four an hour. They may last for anything from a few seconds to several minutes.

They vary in intensity too. Some women experience just a mild blush – indeed, a few have said that they find it rather becoming. But most women feel it is like a hot flush creeping up from the chest to the throat, to the face and right up to the top of the head. Some say it is preceded by a feeling of tension or tingling, others find themselves suddenly suffused with no warning at all. For some the flush is followed by sweating (the body's normal and healthy reaction to over-heating), others experience just a cold sweat and don't flush at all, in fact, they may turn very pale. If a woman sweats a lot, she may subsequently feel cold and even begin to shiver, especially if her clothes have become soaked.

Night sweating

Some women suffer particularly from these symptoms at night. They wake up to find themselves suddenly unbearably hot and struggling to throw off the bed clothes, only then to break out into a cold sweat, followed by shivering. Others wake up already drenched in sweat, sometimes to the point where they have to change not only their night clothes but their bedding as well. Night sweating is probably the most unpleasant form of this symptom, and if it happens very frequently and is very severe, the woman will also begin to suffer from lack of sleep, which may in turn bring exhaustion, irritability, lack of concentration and even depression.

Hormone Replacement Therapy (HRT)

If you are really plagued by these flushes and sweatings, you should certainly consult your doctor, who may prescribe hormone tablets for a while. Since the symptom is probably caused by the drop of the oestrogen level in the blood, to which the body has not yet adjusted, it can be counteracted by replacing the hormones (progesterone is nowadays almost always given in conjunction with oestrogen, as this has been found to be medically safer). This is known as Hormone Replacement Therapy (HRT).

Such tablets must only be taken under medical supervision, as a lot has still to be learned about Hormone Replacement Therapy; it is not the philosopher's stone and cure for aging that it was once hailed to be. However, it is a useful treatment when such help is really needed – a teacher, for instance, felt she had been close to a breakdown until her doctor decided to give her hormone treatment, because she just could not face her class of teenagers while having constant 'overwhelming' flushes. Most doctors in any case will probably only prescribe the treatment for a limited period until the body has found its new hormonal balance. Some doctors are however understandably still very reluctant to make use of HRT, so if you feel strongly that you need the help it could give but your doctor does not want to prescribe it, you could ask for a second opinion. Your doctor will probably suggest that you see a gynaecologist, preferably perhaps a woman. If your GP is not helpful, however, visit your nearest NHS Menopause Clinic.

Coping with flushes

While you cannot do anything to prevent flushes and sweating, you can do quite a lot to make them less unpleasant.

CLOTHING AND BEDDING It is better, for instance, to wear loose clothing, and to wear layers of clothes when it is cold, rather than one thick or restricting garment only, so that you can take off one or two when you begin to feel warm. It is also best to wear wool or cotton, which are absorbent materials, rather than synthetic fibres, which can themselves produce sweating. Duvets are easier to throw off in the night than sheets and blankets that are tucked in, although sheets and blankets can be removed in layers, and it is also a good idea to have an extra blanket ready if you tend to shiver after sweating. If your night sweats are really heavy, keep a change of clothing and bed linen ready to change without fuss.

DIET is an important factor. It is better not to eat too much spicy or highly seasoned food, which causes flushing even without benefit of the menopause, and so does alcohol, which also dilates the blood vessels. If you suffer very badly from flushes, you should really avoid alcohol altogether. The same is true of caffeine – remember that it is present not just in coffee, but also in tea (though not in herbal teas), cola drinks and in chocolate. You should restrict your salt intake too, as salt increases the body's water retention, which may help to trigger off flushes, and too much sugar should also be avoided, as swings in the level of blood sugar may be another contributory factor. If your flushes bother you sufficiently, you will certainly find it worth monitoring them to see which of these items you would do

Have a look in the mirror next time you have a hot flush. You may be pleasantly surprised at how little it actually shows.

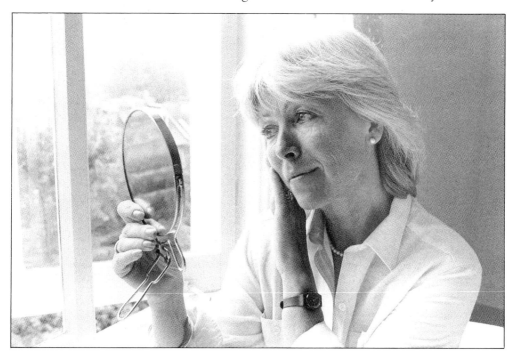

well to avoid, at least for a time.

VITAMINS are vital to your general well-being at all times, and we will be talking more about their necessity in a later chapter (see page 60). But there is some evidence that vitamin E can help to counter-act hot flushes. In a research project in America, 50 per cent of women who took a vitamin E supplement found that their flushes became less intense. (Vitamin E has to be taken in supplement form as it is difficult to take in a lot with ordinary food.)

EXERCISE AND RELAXATION Exercise, which improves circulation, can help too, especially as it also increases natural sweating (see p.66). It seems that women with poor circulation, and those who do not sweat easily, suffer more from hot flushes. Exercise also helps us to relax (see p.67); some women find that they are more likely to have a flush if they are tense or anxious, so exercise and relaxation will help to minimize the problem.

While all these strategies will help, most of us still have to go through a period when hot flushes come and go. When they do, it is no use to try to fight them off: it can't be done, and anyway, fighting only increases tension which in turn exaggerates the symptoms we experience. 'Go with' the flush, let the wave of heat flow over you and recede again, while you relax and breathe deeply (see p.72): remember that most flushes only last for a matter of seconds, or a very few minutes at the most. And finally, don't be embarrassed if you have a flush while you are in company; you can always explain what is happening to friends if you find that talking about it puts you more at your ease, but in any case, even though you may feel that you have turned a deep beetroot red, most people will probably not even be aware that anything is amiss.

The breasts

There is generally an unavoidable loss of breast tissue at this time. The breasts generally shrink a little, become less firm and may begin to sag. Although there are no muscles in the breasts themselves, keeping generally fit, maintaining good posture (see p.68) and, most important, wearing a well-fitting bra, can improve your overall shape.

The vagina

There are also changes in the vagina as we grow older. The outer lips become a little less plump, and as the level of oestrogen in the blood diminishes, the inner lips become paler and pink, rather than purple, and there may be some thinning of the pubic hairs. The inner walls of the vagina also shrink a little and lose some of their elasticity, and the mucous membranes that line the vaginal passage become thinner and smoother, with fewer bumps and ridges. These are natural changes, of which we may be barely aware, but occasionally they can lead to some minor problems.

Because the vaginal walls have shrunk a little and become less elastic, together with the fact that they may be slower to exude their natural lubricant, intercourse can become uncomfortable, at least for a while. You can usually overcome this difficulty by taking a little longer in the build-up to intercourse, so that the vagina has had time to produce the necessary lubrication before the penis enters (see p.39). If the problem persists, you may like to use some external lubricant, such as KY jelly, or a body or massage gel, preferably unscented. Natural vegetable or fruit oils are probably the best. Pelvic floor exercises (see page 117) will also help to maintain the elasticity of the pelvic floor and the vagina.

The best exercise of all is continued sexual activity. If intercourse goes on being uncomfortable, don't choose abstinence, but go and see your doctor, who may prescribe a hormone cream to use for a while. This helps to thicken the membranes of the vaginal wall and make them less sensitive, but it should only be used under medical supervision probably for a short period only, as the tissues of the vagina readily absorb the oestrogen, and there is a slight risk that cancerous cells could develop.

Vaginal infections

Because the inner lining of the vagina has become thinner and less moist, it is also more vulnerable to any slight scratch or tear and to infections, which can cause burning or itching and also make intercourse uncomfortable. In mild cases it may be sufficient to take great care with hygiene: to wear only cotton next to the skin and no nylon tights, and to use only unscented soaps and no detergents when washing your underwear. It may also help to cut out sugar from your diet, as a sugar-rich diet can reduce the acidity of the vagina, which normally prevents harmful bacteria from developing. Some women find that not only eating plenty of yogurt but also using natural unsweetened yogurt in a vaginal douche, or introducing yogurt, undiluted, into the vagina with an applicator, helps to maintain its necessary acidity.

If in spite of these precautions you still have burning or itching, or a vaginal discharge, do go and see your doctor. The changes in the vagina which make it particularly vulnerable to infections at this time mean that it is possible for even the most faithfully monogamous couple to develop thrush. These minute organisms which may have been harboured in the man's genitals quite harmlessly up to now can suddenly cause irritation and infection. This should not be ignored and can usually be treated quite easily with antibiotics.

These are the major physical changes that take place in all women's bodies during the menopause. I remember many years ago returning home late one evening to find my husband and young teenage daughter (who should have been long since in bed) sharing a bottle of wine. They were celebrating the fact that her first period had started that evening. It is a pity that there is no one moment that marks the end of the climacteric so that we could have a similar celebration: it is after all a difficult passage, safely negotiated.

SOME SPECIFIC PROBLEMS

As we saw in the previous chapter, there are normal physical changes that take place during the climacteric and as part of the aging process to which all women have to adapt. There are also others which are not inevitable, but with which many women will have to cope to a greater or lesser degree.

If the list that follows seems formidable, remember that these are specific problems, none of which need necessarily affect you. However, it is important to understand what can happen in your body as the years pass and what difficulties you may encounter. Forewarned is forearmed, and many of these conditions can be prevented; where prevention is not possible, there are often ways of minimizing the extent of the discomfort or distress. Making sure that we understand as much as a lay person can is part of the process of taking responsibility for ourselves, and the better informed we are, the better we can make use of, or, if necessary, campaign for such preventive measures and medical help as are available.

Osteoporosis

Osteoporosis is a stealthy disease from which a woman may suffer for years before becoming aware of it. It is distressing and potentially dangerous, yet it has not always had the publicity that it deserves.

What is osteoporosis?

The bones, like every other part of the body, die off and replace themselves steadily throughout life; in fact, during childhood and youth, while we are still growing, and the active years of early adulthood that follow, the bones renew themselves completely every seven years. As we grow older, the rate of replacement diminishes, and after the age of 35 we lose a very small proportion of our bone mass, probably about half a per cent, each year.

Osteoporosis, however, is a condition where the loss of bone mass is abnormally high, and, as the name implies, the bones become porous, fragile and hence brittle. The result is that they

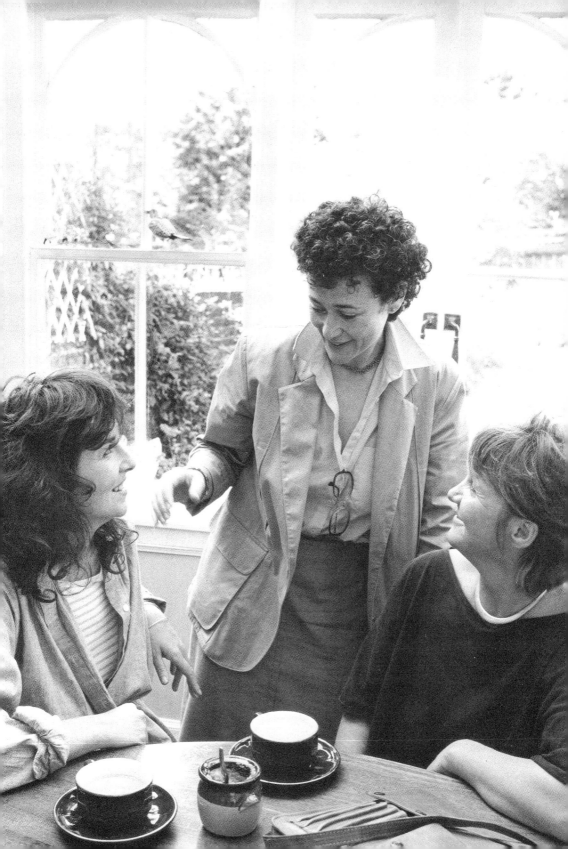

fracture easily, especially the wrist bones, femur and hips, and while the fractures themselves are not fatal, the complications that can set in as a result may be. Think how often you hear of an elderly lady dying of pneumonia after fracturing her hip in a fall. The condition can also affect the spine. The vertebrae may be fractured or simply collapse, and the woman suffer from a curved spine with severe back pain, developing the so-called 'dowager's hump'.

Osteoporosis affects women much more commonly, and much earlier, than men. The bones are the depository of more than 90 per cent of the body's calcium, and they 'sacrifice' it to other parts of the body when needed. If a woman is not careful about her diet, she commonly suffers some loss of calcium during pregnancy or while breastfeeding, for instance. As men have larger bones on average, and do not have the same demands on their bodies from child-bearing, the loss of bone mass is proportionately less for them as they grow older. For women who may have depleted their calcium store earlier in life, the loss of bone mass can be very serious.

Osteoporosis and the menopause

The hormonal changes that take place during the menopause can also have a direct effect on the bones. The older we get, the more calcium we need to maintain our bone structure, but there appears to be a link between the level of oestrogen in the blood and the bones' ability to take up calcium. As the oestrogen level drops during the menopausal years there is a particular danger for women of osteoporosis setting in without any apparent warning signs.

Preventing osteoporosis

While some loss of bone mass is inevitable, osteoporosis is not. It is a disease which can be prevented, and nutrition and exercise are the best prophylactics.

Diet

An adequate supply of calcium is vital. It is particularly important to watch your calcium intake in the very early years of the menopause, and even before it has begun, so that the bones are in good health during this time. The best sources of calcium are low fat milk and yogurt, and cheese, particularly Swiss cheese, canned fish such as salmon and sardines, and dark green leafy vegetables. Alcohol and caffeine can impair the body's ability to take up the calcium, and so does too much phosphorous in the diet, so it is better to eat less salt and less meat, especially red meat, which are all rich in phosphorous. In fact, some studies have shown that women in this age group who have been vegetarians for many years have twice the bone mass of women of the same age who eat meat. Fortunately, our bodies know best, if we can only know how to listen to them, and many of us find that we actually want less meat as we grow older. There is also new evidence that it is important not to become *too* thin, since metabolic activity in the subcutaneous fat actually helps to prevent osteoporosis.

Taking exercise

Exercise can also do a lot to prevent osteoporosis. Bones need regular exercise and stress to remain healthy (see page 66); exercise is a vital stimulus to the bones to rebuild themselves. Even if osteoporosis has already set in, appropriate exercise, properly supervised, can still help to prevent the condition from deteriorating. Strenuous exercise should be avoided at all costs, but the gentle movements of activities, such as walking or playing golf, are particularly beneficial.

Treating osteoporosis

While keeping fit and healthy through proper diet and regular exercise are the best preventives, there is no cure and no way of reversing osteoporosis: once the bones have deteriorated, it is impossible to rebuild them. The only hope is to prevent this disease from progressing further. Unfortunately it is also very difficult to diagnose; a woman may not know she is suffering from it for many years, until the time when her bones are already so brittle that they easily fracture. Nor is it known what makes someone prone to the disease, although there are some indications that there is an hereditary link, and also that women who have a very early menopause (either natural or surgically induced by hysterectomy) or women who have not had children, are more likely to suffer from it.

When osteoporosis sets in during the menopause, Hormone Replacement Therapy (HRT: see p.16) can be used to help arrest the weakening of the bones. Women who have reason to believe that they are likely to suffer from osteoporosis may well decide to take this option. However, it is important to start the treatment very early in the climacteric, and it must be continued for many years, at least until the age of 65 or thereabouts. If it is stopped too soon, the bones will deteriorate just as if the hormones had never been taken. Since hormones will only help the bones to take up the necessary calcium, a proper diet and exercise remain vital and the doctor will probably also recommend calcium and vitamin supplements.

High blood pressure (hypertension)

High blood pressure is another health hazard for everyone over 40, and, like osteoporosis, it can go undetected until it is almost too late. Our blood pressure rises and falls in time with the heart beat – it is greatest when the heart contracts (the systolic level) and least when it relaxes (the diastolic level). These pressure levels are expressed as 'systolic over diastolic', for instance, 140/80 or 150/85, either of which may be normal for an adult. When the level rises above these figures, there is a danger of stroke, heart failure and thrombosis, especially if the body is subjected to shock or sudden vigorous exercise.

Causes of hypertension

Several factors can contribute to an increase in blood pressure. Hypertension runs in families, just like red hair or blue eyes, so it pays to be vigilant if any close members of your family have suffered from heart disease or stroke. Other contributory factors include being overweight, eating poorly (especially too many fatty foods,

Gentle exercise reduces muscle tension and can help you relax.

salt and refined sugar), smoking, drinking too much alcohol, and emotional and physical stress.

High blood pressure may cause headaches and blurred vision, but usually there are few warning signals. Regular medical check-ups twice a year by your doctor or at a 'well woman' clinic are therefore very important.

Preventing hypertension

Try to keep your weight down to a reasonable level, and combine a healthy diet (see p.59) with regular exercise (see p.64). If you smoke, cut it down and, if possible, give it up altogether. Learning how to cope with stress is one of the best preventive measures: stress makes the muscles tighten involuntarily, constricting the blood vessels, which can raise the blood pressure. Gentle rhythmic exercise with correct breathing (see p.72), massage and above all relaxation (see p.119) are all extremely beneficial in helping to rid you of muscle tension.

If your blood pressure rises

If you are suffering from hypertension you may be advised to lose weight, to stop smoking and to restrict your salt intake. You should also stop taking the contraceptive pill. Relaxation is particularly helpful (see p.119), especially if the rise in blood pressure has been exacerbated by emotional or physical stress. In some cases, the doctor may prescribe drugs, but if so, do ask him to explain why these are necessary, and for how long you will need to take them. Ask also about the possibility of any side effects so that you are prepared for them, and whether the drugs are likely to have an effect on your level of sexual desire.

Gentle exercise is probably beneficial in that it reduces overall muscle tension and helps you to relax properly afterwards, but strenuous sports such as squash or aerobic dancing should be avoided at all costs. You should always check with your doctor before embarking on any form of exercise, however apparently innocuous (see p.67).

Diabetes

Diabetes is a disorder of the body's metabolism which sometimes affects men and women in late middle age. In this age group it is generally caused by the body's inability to respond to insulin, which means that sugar and starches are not properly processed. The excess sugar in the blood stream is passed out directly in urine, so that once diabetes is suspected, it is easy to diagnose through a simple urine test. Like hypertension, there can be an hereditary tendency to diabetes, so you should have regular urine tests if there is any history of diabetes in your family.

Diabetes eventually interferes with the metabolizing of fats and proteins, so if left untreated can lead to serious complications involving the blood vessels, kidneys, heart, eyes and nerve-endings.

Signs and symptoms

Your doctor may suspect you are suffering from diabetes if you have any or a combination of the following symptoms: if you have excessive thirst; if you need to pass urine frequently, both day and

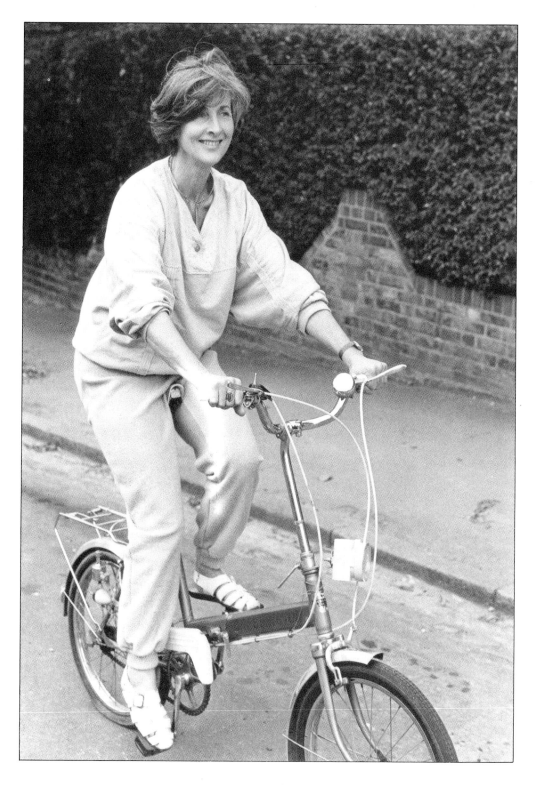

night; if you have an associated irritation from an infection around the vulva; and if you are overweight.

Preventive measures

There is a correlation between overweight and diabetes, though it is not yet clear whether the obesity is cause or effect; in any case it pays to keep your weight down within reasonable limits (see p.58). Stress may unmask diabetes in susceptible people, so good diet and regular exercise, combined with relaxation (see p.119), may help to avoid it.

Treating diabetes

Mid-life diabetes can usually be controlled by a combination of diet and drugs, and often by the former alone. A reduced intake of refined sugars is essential, which can only be beneficial to your overall well-being (see p.59). If you become a diabetic at this stage in your life, you are very unlikely to need insulin injections.

Vaginal prolapse

Vaginal prolapse occurs when the vaginal walls weaken and collapse into the vaginal cavity, allowing the uterus, the rectum, the bladder and sometimes the urethra, to drop down and even to protrude. Uterine prolapse may cause discomfort on intercourse; if the rectum, bladder or urethra have dropped, there will be discomfort on opening the bowels or passing urine.

Types of prolapse

Lack of muscle tone or damage to the vaginal walls during childbirth, combined with hormonal changes in the menopause, cause the walls of the vagina to collapse. This allows adjacent organs to bulge or protrude into the vaginal cavity.

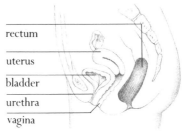

rectum

uterus

bladder

urethra

vagina

The pelvic organs in their usual position.

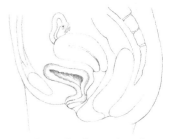

Urethrocele The urethra (the tube through which urine is passed from the bladder) bulges against the front of the vagina.

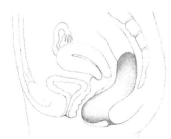

Rectocele The rectum pushes against the back of the vagina, causing severe discomfort when opening the bowels.

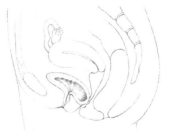

Cystocele The bladder pushes against the upper front wall of the vagina, causing 'stress incontinence' and cystitis.

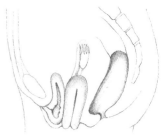

Uterine prolapse The uterus and cervix slip down into the vaginal cavity. This is the most common form of prolapse.

Injury to the pelvic floor muscles during childbirth, or allowing them to remain slack and weak afterwards, are the commonest causes of prolapse. Lack of oestrogen following the menopause also causes the pelvic organs to shrink and the muscles can lose further tone.

Suspecting prolapse

Tiredness, backache and a dragging feeling of 'something coming down' are the usual signs of prolapse. 'Stress incontinence' – passing urine when coughing, laughing or sneezing – or a discharge or bleeding from the vagina due to ulceration of the prolapse, are also symptoms.

Treating prolapse

If you suspect you may have a prolapse, do not delay in consulting your doctor, as early prolapse can be reversed by physiotherapy and exercise. In serious cases, abdominal surgery to repair the injured tissues, or hysterectomy (see below), are the most usual forms of treatment. While exercise to strengthen the pelvic floor muscles is the best preventive measure (see p.117), after surgery exercise should only be done on the advice of the doctor and physiotherapist, since the timing and type of exercise will depend on the precise surgery that has been undertaken.

Sometimes a pessary consisting of a polythene ring can be inserted to support the dropped organs. This must be checked every four to six months, but if fitted properly causes no discomfort and does not interfere with sexual intercourse.

Hysterectomy

Hysterectomy is the medical name given to the operation for the removal of the uterus and some of its associated reproductive organs. Most hysterectomies are performed on women over the age of 50. In the United States it has been estimated that more than a quarter of all women over 50 have had a hysterectomy; in Britain the incidence is not so high, but still high enough for us to need to inform ourselves very clearly what the circumstances are under which we might need to have this operation. A hysterectomy is a major operation, with important physical and emotional consequences, and no one should agree to undergo it without being fully convinced that it is necessary.

Types of hysterectomy

There are two main types of hysterectomy. When the uterus, the cervix, the fallopian tubes and the ovaries are all removed through an incision in the abdominal wall the operation is known as a 'complete' hysterectomy. It is known as 'total' when only the uterus, together with the cervix, are removed through the abdominal wall, or sometimes through an incision in the vagina (this operation leaves no external scars). Occasionally a 'sub-total' hysterectomy is also performed, which leaves behind the cervix as well as the ovaries and the fallopian tubes.

Reasons for the operation

The most common reasons for which doctors recommend hysterectomy are cancer (or the presence of pre-cancerous cells) in the

Types of hysterectomy

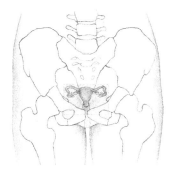

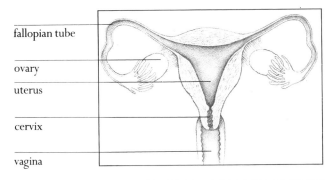

fallopian tube

ovary

uterus

cervix

vagina

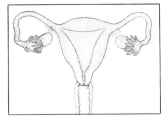

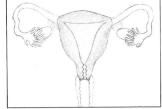

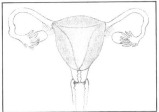

Complete hysterectomy: here the uterus, cervix, ovaries and fallopian tubes are all removed.

Total hysterectomy: in this operation, only the uterus and cervix are removed.

Sub-total hysterectomy: here the uterus alone is removed, leaving the cervix in place.

cervix, uterus, fallopian tubes or ovaries; large fibroids; severe pelvic infection; or when a woman continues to haemorrhage despite hormone treatment (see p.14).

Cancer

Cervical cancer, which, next to breast cancer, is the most common form of the disease in women, can be easily detected in the early stages, so the most sensible precaution to take is to have regular smear tests. However, cervical cancer becomes less of a risk as we get older, while the incidence of uterine cancer increases with age: 75 per cent of uterine cancer patients are over 50. The early warning signs of this are bleeding or spotting between periods, or after the periods have ceased, and such bleeding should always be investigated by a doctor. Even though it is very natural to be frightened if you suspect you may have cancer, don't adopt an ostrich policy – putting your head in the sand is the worst thing you can do. All cancers are best treated as soon as they are diagnosed, and the sooner they are diagnosed, the less radical the treatment is likely to have to be.

Fibroids

Fibroids can cause heavy bleeding, but as they generally shrink during the menopause (see p.14), it may be best to leave them unless they cause very severe discomfort. Some fibroids are so large however that they cause pressure on the bladder or intestinal tract, and their removal may be necessary. It is often possible to shell the growths out of the uterus with a spoon-like instrument in a minor

Fibroids

Fibroids are non-malignant tumours in the uterine wall.

1 Small fibroids usually cause little trouble, shrinking at the menopause.

2 Fibroids which grow inwards can cause heavy bleeding, perhaps necessitating a hysterectomy.

3 Fibroids that grow outwards may press against organs such as the rectum or bladder.

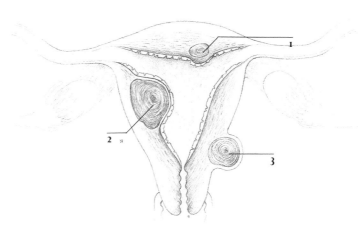

operation, called a myomectomy. This is infinitely preferable to a hysterectomy, which should not be necessary unless the doctor has reason to believe that the growths may be pre-cancerous or because they have been causing such heavy bleeding that your life is in danger. If pre-cancerous growths are suspected it is usually possible to do a biopsy first to establish whether a hysterectomy is really necessary.

Pelvic infections and haemorrhaging

Even very severe pelvic infections can often be treated by massive doses of antibiotics, and this should certainly be tried before anything as serious as a hysterectomy is contemplated. Very heavy bleeding or haemorrhaging should also be extensively investigated before a hysterectomy is performed unless the bleeding is quite uncontrollable and the woman's life is at risk (see Fibroids above).

Questioning the need for hysterectomy

Obviously there are many instances where there are good reasons for doctors to advise a hysterectomy, and often a woman's life can be saved by it. But unfortunately the medical profession, still largely dominated by men, has in the past taken a rather callously non-chalant attitude to the operation: perhaps it has been hard for male gynaecologists to understand how important the uterus remains to a woman, even when she is past the child-bearing age.

If you have been advised to have a hysterectomy, it is important to assert yourself in requesting a full discussion and explanation from your doctor. This may be quite hard to do, especially when you are probably feeling upset at the time. You are also entitled to ask for, and if necessary to insist upon, a second opinion. Where alternative treatment is a possibility, consider it carefully, and always, except in cases of emergency, take the time to discuss the options fully with your partner, family and any friends who have been in a similar situation.

You should also discuss with the doctor or surgeon how complete the hysterectomy is going to be; all too often surgeons perform a complete hysterectomy where a partial ('total') one might be adequate, arguing that this will save possible trouble later on. However, if the ovaries can be saved they should be, as they continue to affect the body's hormone production even after the menopause is over.

Once you have explored the alternatives and are satisfied that a hysterectomy is the right course, you will be able to go into the operation in the best frame of mind. It is always a major operation, and after the week or so in hospital you will need to convalesce for at least five to six weeks and it is vital that you allow yourself that time.

Physical and mental recovery

And the convalescence will not be only a physical one. A hysterectomy is a kind of bereavement: the woman has lost a very vital part of herself, and she will need time, and sustained loving care from her partner, family and friends, to come to terms with the loss. Feelings of loss or depression can go on for as long as six months or a year, but although some grief is inevitable, it has been found that women who were convinced that their hysterectomy was essential recover better, and are less likely to suffer from depression later, than those who had the operation without such understanding or acceptance. Being able to talk about your feelings to a sympathetic listener – your partner, a friend or a counsellor – is probably the greatest help.

In most cases the operation is entirely successful, and once fully recovered, the woman returns to a normal life. Usually she will feel much better than before, since the debilitating symptoms which had previously drained her energies have now been removed. These may well have affected her sex life as well, and although many women worry that their sex lives will suffer from having had a hysterectomy, the opposite is more often the case.

Breast cancer and mastectomy

Breast cancer is probably the disease that women fear most, and rightly so, as it remains the leading cause of death from cancer in women, with the incidence rising as we get older. While we cannot prevent it, we can do a great deal ourselves to control it. As with cervical cancer, early diagnosis is the vital key, and it is such a simple procedure that we should be able to seek medical help immediately a lump is detected. Breast cancer is an absolutely curable disease if caught early enough, so regular breast examinations are a must for all women whatever their age, but especially for those of us over the age of 40.

Breast examination

It is a very simple procedure, which you can do yourself; the technique is described opposite. It is important that you examine your breasts regularly, at least every three months. Certain women are in a high risk group, and should examine themselves monthly. If your mother or sister has had breast cancer, if you have had benign

How to examine your breasts

You should examine your breasts at least every 3 months. Consult your doctor at once if you find anything unusual.

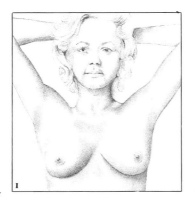

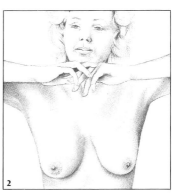

1 Remove your clothes and sit or stand straight in front of a mirror. Look at the shape of your breasts carefully, noting any changes in shape or level of the breasts and nipples. Check there is no discharge from the nipple or change of skin texture. Raise your arms above your head and look for swelling or puckering.

2 Join your hands in front of your chin, elbows raised. Lean towards the mirror and look at each breast for anything unusual in outline and texture, or position of the nipple.

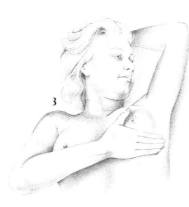

3 Lie down in a comfortable position, perhaps in the bath. Feel each breast in turn as follows, using the left hand for the right breast and vice versa. Using the flat of your hand, fingers straight and together, slide your hand over the breast above the nipple starting at the armpit. Press in to feel for lumps, but not so hard that you dull the sensation. Do not pinch the breast. Repeat the action for the area below the nipple.

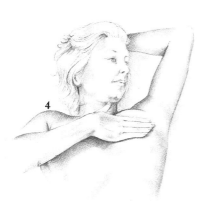

4 Keeping your hand flat, slide it across the nipple from armpit to centre, again feeling for lumps.

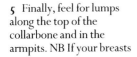

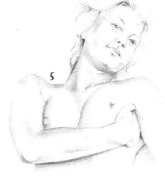

5 Finally, feel for lumps along the top of the collarbone and in the armpits. NB If your breasts are very full, you may need to support them gently with your free hand during the examination.

lumps in the breast in the past, if you have not had children or had them very late in life, then you come into this category .

Finding a breast abnormality

If, when you make your regular examination, you detect a lump or bump, hard or soft, any change in the shape of the breast or the texture or colour of the skin, if the nipple has become scaly or there is a discharge, see your doctor at once. Remember that the great majority of such growths are benign, but just in case it is not, the sooner it is dealt with, the better.

Your doctor will probably act very promptly and send you straight away to a surgeon for further examination. This does not mean that he thinks the lump is malignant, but just that he must, responsibly, treat all symptoms as though they are, until proved innocent. Remember that time is of the essence here, and that if you should have a malignant lump, the smaller it is, the more easily it can be excised.

Diagnosing the lump

The first step is to ascertain the nature of the lump. The surgeon will either 'aspirate' or do a needle biopsy. This is not a painful procedure, and will probably be sufficient for making a diagnosis, though an x-ray, or mammograph, may also need to be taken (these are not done as routinely in England as they are in the US). If neither of these tests prove conclusive, the surgeon may decide to perform a biopsy or a lumpectomy, that is, to remove a part or the whole of the lump for examination. This is only a minor operation, but it should be clearly understood between you and the surgeon that this is all that will be done: in the past women were sometimes asked to agree to having a mastectomy at the same time if it should prove to

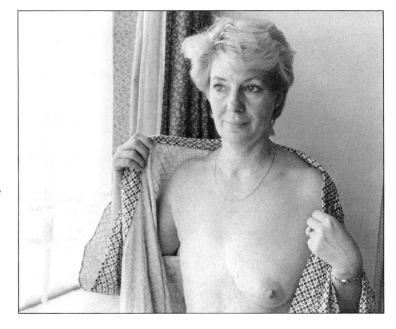

Coming to terms with the sense of loss after a mastectomy is often the most painful part of the whole experience, but a sensitive and loving partner can give the greatest help towards recovery.

be advisable. This is not good practice, and you should not agree to it.

What happens next

If the diagnosis does prove positive, the surgeon and your doctor should discuss with you what the options are. Obviously you will listen to their advice, but the better informed and the more involved you are with the decision, the better you will be able to accept the treatment and any after-effects.

Where the cancer has not spread, a lumpectomy, or removal of the lump itself, with the immediately surrounding tissues and possibly some of the lymph nodes, may be sufficient. In other cases, and where a lump has already grown too big, a part or whole of the breast may have to be removed, often preceded and followed by radiotherapy. For older women, particularly those who completed their menopause at least five years before, hormone therapy alone has often been found to be effective in eradicating the cancer.

If there is to be an operation, make sure the surgeon explains exactly how much he intends to remove and why, so that you can begin to prepare yourself and the extent of the operation does not come as too much of a shock. But do not consent to total removal of

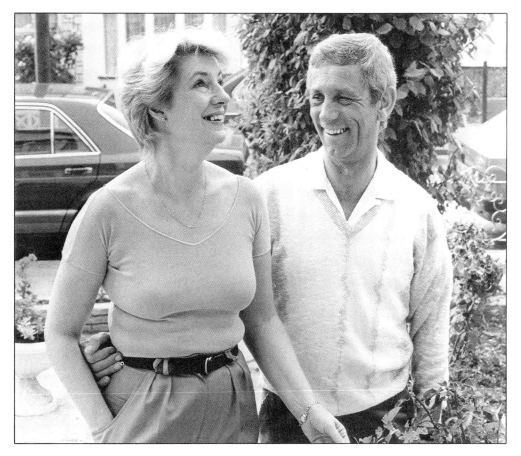

the breast or to the 'Halstead mastectomy' (in which not only the whole breast but also the pectoral muscle and armpit lymph nodes are removed), without being given very good reason and time to think about it. You may want to get a second opinion as well. Recent research has shown that such a radical and mutilating operation does not usually have better results than a simple or partial mastectomy, combined with radiation treatment.

Ask to be told also what the after-effects are likely to be, so that at least you will not be frightened that something has gone wrong if you are in pain, or feeling nauseous. The degree of post-operative 'discomfort', as the euphemism goes, varies considerably, both with the type of operation and also from one woman to the next, and some find that they still have sharp pains as well as dull aching, not just where the operation was, but in all the surrounding areas, for weeks and even months after the operation. Gentle and appropriate exercise as advised by the hospital physiotherapist can be very helpful.

Coping with the sense of loss

For many women the sense of loss is the worst part of the mastectomy, and it is not unusual for a woman to become quite deeply depressed afterwards. Not only has she had the scare of learning that she has cancer, but she has lost a part of her body that is deeply precious to her. While the womb is the seat of female reproductive capacity, and so symbolizes femininity, the breasts seem to symbolize our sexuality, and we are even more intimately identified with them.

Although she may be making a good and quick recovery physically, a woman often feels the emotional pain very deeply, and she will need an opportunity to express this. Few doctors or nursing staff are trained to deal with this distress, and her family and friends may also find her pain too hard to bear. Some, but all too few, hospitals provide counsellors specifically to help women through this period; where this is not provided it is helpful to find someone, a friend or a professional, who can allow you to express your sorrow without being overwhelmed by it themselves. (See also p.124.)

Some women worry about their appearance after such an operation. However there are many good prostheses which can be matched to your size and shape and which can even be worn when swimming or sunbathing. Only when completely naked is there no hiding the loss of the breast and the scars. This is often the hardest part to come to terms with, and many women find it difficult to believe that they can still be sexually attractive, and that their partners can still love and desire them. This is where reassurance from a gently loving husband or lover can usually provide the best help to recovery (see p.42).

Mood swings

'Involutional Melancholia' is what doctors used to call it, as though women in the menopause suffered from some kind of degenerative psychiatric disorder. 'Mood swings' is what we tend to call it now, though that too is a misnomer, since few of us actually experience great elation during this transition period. Many women do suffer from some degree of depression, or at the least irritability, anxiety, chronic tiredness, headaches, inability to concentrate and insomnia – all of them aspects of depression.

There may be many good reasons for this, both internal and external, physical and emotional, and since our minds and bodies are so delicately interlinked, it is often hard to know what is the cause, and in which direction we should look for help.

Usually a great deal is going on in our lives at this time, and many changes taking place. Children are leaving home; our careers may be at their most demanding or we may be suffering from disappointments at work; husbands too are at the peak of their careers or else trying to come to terms with retirement; parents are aged or dying and need a lot of help and nurturing. Our old roles are slipping away, new ones have to be forged (see p.46). All this can quite reasonably make us feel angry and perplexed as well as sad.

Meanwhile our bodies too are adjusting to many changes, especially the hormones which are finding their new equilibrium (see p.13). This in turn affects the way we think and feel. Just as in adolescence and after childbirth, the fluctuating hormones produce shifting moods, and just as at those times, it is hard to know how much our moods and anxieties are due to the chemical changes, and how much to the new circumstances of our lives. Indeed, it is pointless to try to make the distinction; we must just accept that mind and body are interdependent parts of our whole being, and try to help ourselves on both fronts.

Expressing your feelings

If you are tired, allow yourself to rest. If you are angry, say so, don't bottle it up until you burst. Talking about how you feel almost always helps, especially with a friend or a group of women who are going through similar experiences. It helps to know that you are not the only one feeling like this: it gives you permission to feel what you feel, and exploring aloud what your feelings are often also helps to dissipate them. Once you have said out loud to someone who really listens that you are angry or sad, you will probably find that some of the heat has gone out of the feeling.

A healthy diet helps too (see p.59), whereas another cup of coffee, another gin and tonic, another cigarette or another chocolate biscuit, do not. And exercise can also be a great help (see p.69). Vigorous movement actually releases beneficial hormones, and anyway, it is hard to feel depressed while running, jumping or skipping!

If nothing seems to help, and you continue to feel really depressed, then do go and see your doctor, who may well prescribe hormone therapy for a while, until the hormones have settled to their new equilibrium.

SEX AND SEXUALITY

Attitudes to sexuality

We are sexual beings from the moment we are born to the day we die, and to deny that is to deny an important part of ourselves.

Men have always known this, and have celebrated their sexuality. Small boys proudly display and compare their penises, young men boast of their conquests. Infant boys sometimes have erections within hours of birth, and we all have an affectionate admiration for men like Picasso, who continued to be joyously sexual well into his 80s and 90s.

But for women, sexuality has been a more difficult issue. Small girls, while encouraged to be flirtatious and winsome, are still not supposed to be sexually aware. Most of us now in our 40s and 50s were brought up with the confusing message that sex is not for nice girls; yet sex is beautiful and should be kept for the man you love and marry.

Meanwhile, over the last twenty years, sex has suddenly become a public issue, and all matters sexual are subjects for open and explicit discussion. This in turn has brought its own constraints, so that at various stages of life, women may feel under subtle pressure either to deny their sexuality, or to pretend to a more active sex life than they actually have. Teenagers frequently suffer from the latter, the middle-aged from the former. Sex tends to be presented by the media as the prerogative of the young and the beautiful. As a result, young girls may find themselves forced into being sexually active before they are ready to cope with the powerful emotions that are unleashed, while middle-aged and elderly women are supposed not to have sexual needs.

Sex and maturity

We have probably all unconsciously subscribed to this attitude in our time. Which of us cannot remember the conviction that we were the first to discover the delights of sex, newly minted, and also that surely our parents didn't still 'do it' at their age? And, if we are

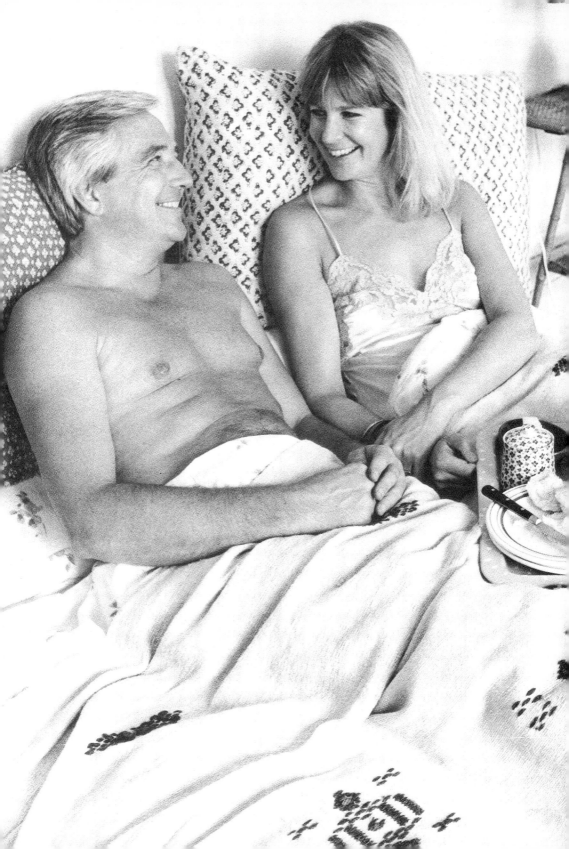

honest, we probably still find it hard to imagine anyone twenty or more years older than ourselves making love.

Now, thanks to research done on both sides of the Atlantic, but notably in the United States by William Kinsey in the 1950s and Shere Hite in the 1970s, we know that given the opportunity, men and women remain sexually active all their lives. And, in contrast to men, women only reach their full sexual awareness and potential in their late 30s or early 40s. While men reach the peak of their sexual capacity at the age of 17 or 18, after which their capacity declines gradually but steadily, women enjoy sex more as they get older. Their responsiveness is at its height in their late 30s and early 40s, and only declines very slowly thereafter.

This can be good news for men and women alike. Where young men are often impetuous, too quick to enter and too quick to climax, leaving their partners barely aroused, the older man takes longer to have an erection and he has probably also learned to control his ejaculation, so the couple have more time to enjoy a slower build-up to intercourse. 'Age slows sex down,' said a 53-year-old man in Shere Hite's survey on male sexuality, 'but this isn't bad. Both partners enjoy a higher level of pleasure.' And another: 'I enjoy it more now too because I can stretch the act out longer and enjoy it more. Premature ejaculation is no longer a problem. It's not as frantic an act as it was, I can savour it more.' And a woman who had been married for nearly thirty years told me, 'I used to read about foreplay, but I never really knew what it meant. Now we really "play" together and it's wonderful.'

Meanwhile, just when the man is able to take longer over the sex act, the older woman is more quickly aroused. While young women frequently have difficulty with arousal and reaching orgasm, Masters and Johnson, the American father and mother of sex therapy, found that older women, and especially if they have had children, are much more likely to lubricate easily and to have one or more orgasms during intercourse. 'Nowadays I know that if I just let it happen, I'll probably have an orgasm, and then another, and then perhaps another. I don't have to fight for it any more,' said a woman in her mid 50s.

The advantages of experience

There may be many reasons for this. A couple who have been together for some time are more attuned to one another; an older man may be more skilled in arousing his partner, and if he is not, an older woman is more likely to have the confidence to tell or show him what gives her pleasure. 'I used to think that all that mattered was that he got his pleasure. In my heart of hearts I even believed that it wan't quite nice for women to enjoy sex – that was the climate in which I grew up,' a woman in her late 50s said. 'But nowadays, if I'm with a partner who does not know how to arouse me, I tell him. After all, sex is for mutual pleasure, even though it took me a long time to learn that.'

As children grow older, couples can enjoy more privacy, with less fear of interruption, during the day as well as at night. 'I am enjoying sex more in my 40s than I did in my 30s; I enjoyed it more in my 30s than in my 20s,' said one woman in response to Shere Hite's question, How does age affect sex? 'There is a liberating combination of experience, self-knowledge and confidence, and an absence of pregnancy fears.'

There is also an absence of 'performance fears'. Women have probably always known that sex is more than intercourse, and intercourse more than a means of arriving at orgasm. But in earlier years there is often a pressure for a woman to 'achieve' (significant word) orgasm, as much for the man's sake, who may otherwise feel he has failed, as for herself. As couples get older, making love without the climax of orgasm does not have to feel like failure. Men and women alike can enjoy closeness and intimacy for their own sake: stroking, caressing and embracing can be for mutual comfort and delight, and do not necessarily have to lead to intercourse each time.

Sex and the menopause

The shift in the balance of libido between men and women can also be of mutual benefit. Whereas a young man's frequent and urgent need for sex can cause problems for young couples, this biological urge diminishes with age in men, while a woman's appetite for sex increases as she becomes more skilled and is more often satisfied – it 'grows by what it feeds on'. And in theory at least, the menopause should not interfere with this. To quote Helen Singer Kaplan, the highly regarded American authority on sex and sex therapy: 'From a purely physiological standpoint, libido should theoretically increase at menopause, because the action of the woman's androgens [hormones which increase libido], which is not materially affected by menopause, is now unopposed by oestrogen.'

In practice, however, women do sometimes experience a loss of libido during the menopause. This may be due to tiredness, especially if she loses a lot of sleep because of night sweating, or to depression. Or it may be because intercourse has become un-comfortable for a while. As we saw in Chapter 1, the walls of the vagina undergo some changes: they become thinner and less elastic, and for a while lubrication may take longer. It is important that you and your partner recognize this as part of the physiological changes taking place, and not as a sign of diminished sexual interest. Explain, if necessary, that if you are not lubricating, it is not because you do not want to make love, but because at this period your body is not responding in the usual way, and you need to spend more time on becoming aroused, before you are ready for intercourse.

In fact, the more frequently and regularly you engage in sexual activity, whether with a partner or by masturbating, the more easily you will lubricate, and the more you exude your own natural lubricant, the healthier your vagina will remain (see p.19). Women in this age group who are not in a regular sexual relationship therefore benefit particularly from masturbation, as very infrequent intercourse can be uncomfortable or downright painful if the vagina remains dry.

As the membranes that line the vagina become thinner, they also become more vulnerable to infection, and so does the urinary tract. This can cause itching or burning, which is no recipe for sexual arousal, and, as we saw earlier, it is important to deal with these problems and not to let them interfere permanently with your sex life.

Keeping sexually active

Remaining sexually active, with or without a partner, also helps to keep the various muscles of the uterus, the pelvic floor and the vagina well toned. The uterine muscles contract involuntarily during orgasm, and exercising the pelvic floor muscles as described on page 117 will in turn enhance your sex life, as well as preventing the tendency to incontinence to which older women are sometimes prone.

Masturbation can be beneficial therefore, as well as being a very good way of releasing sexual tension. While none of us any longer believe the old wives' tales, many of us still do have some inhibitions about masturbation. We don't really like to talk about it – although some brave women have written whole books on the subject (see Bibliography p.124) – and many women who do masturbate wish they didn't. 'I don't know what's wrong with me,' confided a woman in her late 40s, 'but although sex with my husband is better than it's ever been, I still keep on wanting to masturbate. I haven't masturbated like this since my teens, and I'm really ashamed of myself.' There is no need to be ashamed. The fact that she wanted to experience sexual satisfaction even more was a tribute to, not an adverse reflection on, the pleasure she was experiencing with her husband.

For women who do not find it easy to have an orgasm in intercourse, masturbation is particularly important. When trying to help a woman who cannot climax during intercourse, most sex therapists will first make sure she can masturbate herself to orgasm, and if necessary teach her. To quote from *Our Bodies Ourselves* by the Boston Women's Health Collective: 'Masturbation allows us the time and space to explore and experiment with our own bodies. We can learn what fantasies turn us on, what touches arouse and please us, at what tempo and where. We can come to know our own patterns of sexual response. We don't need to worry about a partner's needs and opinions. Then, if and when we choose, we can share our knowledge by telling or showing our partner, by taking his or her hand and guiding it to touch the places we want touched.'

Sex then is not only a life-enhancing pleasure and a wonderful way of expressing love and experiencing closeness, it is also good for us! But although there are no physical reasons why we should not continue to enjoy it all our lives, there are many personal reasons or circumstances that can make it difficult.

Difficulties with sex

Not all of us have partners, and the older we get the more likely we are to be single. Not only do women live longer than men, but when marriages break up in mid-life, it is much more often the husband who remarries, and usually to a younger woman. Of course not all women want to be married or in a permanent partnership: many prefer to have only occasional sexual relationships without long-term ties and obligations. Some deliberately choose celibacy, but others may feel it thrust upon them. Loneliness is hard for most of us to bear, and, once experienced, the closeness we can feel with another person when making love is painfully missed.

If you are alone

We will be talking more about living alone in the next chapter, but it is appropriate here to say that women on their own should not be ashamed to acknowledge their sexual needs. Difficult though it may still be for us now in this age group, younger women have shown us that it is all right for women to take the initiative, in sex as elsewhere. Provided no one is at risk of being hurt, you *can* let a man know that you find him attractive and would like a sexual relationship with him – a mature woman does not have to be a wallflower, passively waiting to be picked, and a mature man will respect her the more for her honesty and guts. Women who are attracted to other women have different cultural conditioning to overcome, especially if they have not had a lesbian relationship before.

Problems for couples

Even if they have been together for a long time, couples too can experience new difficulties. They may have got bored with sex that has just become a routine, or they may be having to adjust to a new imbalance of sexual desire. Just when the woman may be enjoying an upsurge of sexual energy, especially if she has finished with the menopause, the man, as he gets older, needs a longer period between erections, and it is quite usual for a man in his 50s to need at least a day or two before he can make love again. And, as we have seen, most men also become slower to ejaculate. This can be advantageous (see p.38), but it can also lead to difficulties.

Men in middle age

A man who is at the peak of his career may be stretched to the limit of his energies, especially if he also has to work hard to maintain his position in the face of younger colleagues. Alternatively, he may be disappointed that his career has not been more successful, and having to accept the fact that he is not now likely to rise further. He may have experienced a long period of unemployment, or had to come to terms with redundancy or early retirement. All this can affect his sexual responses and needs.

It is not unusual for a man who is feeling dispirited or disappointed in his career to go through a period when he either cannot have or cannot maintain an erection. Such temporary or sporadic impotence is not in itself alarming, though many men take fright at the least hint of losing their potency. The best way that a woman can help her partner is by reassuring him that this is almost certainly only temporary, and that she has every confidence the erections will return. To react angrily, or to feel hurt, rejected or cheated, will only put further strain on him and on the relationship.

The best way to help him to regain his erection is by helping him to relax, with gentle, undemanding sex play. A woman may like to assume the superior position, with the man lying comfortably on his back and she kneeling astride him. She can then gently fondle and stroke the penis, and eventually guide it, even if not fully erect, into the vagina. Once a man has been able to regain an erection, he will be less devastated if the problem recurs.

Losing interest

When one partner in a couple who have had a good sexual relationship suddenly or gradually loses interest in making love, there may be many reasons which need to be aired before the problem can be resolved.

Extra-marital affairs

In order to reassure themselves that their sexual powers are not waning, some men will seek extra-marital affairs, especially with younger women. A woman too, may have a relationship outside the marriage at this stage. An affair, especially with a younger partner, can be very exciting and rejuvenating, and a wonderful reassurance that one is still sexually potent or attractive, but unless it is handled with great delicacy and understanding, can only too easily destroy a marriage.

Drink, smoking, drugs and illness

There could be other reasons for loss of sexual interest. While alcohol can initially remove inhibitions and enhance sexual appetite, too much invariably depresses sexual desire and can produce impotence. Smoking and obesity inhibit sexual response, and so do depression and some drugs, notably those prescribed for hyper-tension and depression. There are also certain illnesses, such as diabetes, of which impotence or loss of libido can be an early warning signal, and if no other explanation fits, you should consult your doctor.

Post-operative shock

When a woman has had a hysterectomy or a mastectomy, she will need a period of physical and emotional recovery before her sexual feelings can flow again (see p.30). Her partner too may be suffering from shock, and also be afraid to touch her in case he causes pain. Initially, the woman will probably just need the reassuring comfort of closeness and caressing, but gradually she will be able to guide her lover, and the couple will have to explore anew how love-making can give pleasure without discomfort. They may have to find new positions; after a mastectomy especially it may be painful for her to lie on the operated side, or to lie on or crouch over her lover. But even if love-making presents new difficulties for a while, to know that she is still desirable can be the most vital aid to her recovery.

Physical problems

Rheumatism, arthritis or back trouble can also affect love-making. If one partner suffers from back pain, it may be time to buy a new bed, with a hard mattress, or you may find it better to use the floor, with plenty of cushions. If the man is suffering with his back, he may find the most comfortable position is for him to sit upright in a chair, with his partner kneeling astride him, supporting herself with the arms of the chair. Rheumatism and arthritis sufferers can often alleviate discomfort with strategically placed cushions under the knees or the small of the back, and they will also need to experiment with different positions, such as those illustrated

A close relationship with a younger partner can be reassuring as well as rejuvenating.

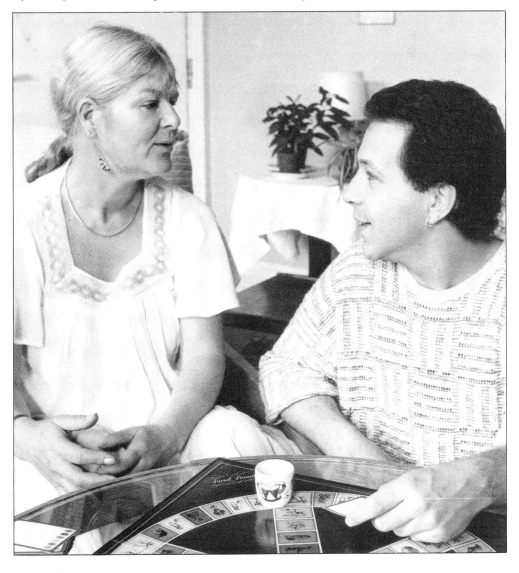

Fantasies

below, to find the one most comfortable for each partner.

As well as overcoming physical difficulties, such experimenting with new positions can also bring new life into what may have become a rather tired routine. Some couples who feel their sex life has become stale also like to use fantasies to inject new excitement. Sharing your fantasies requires a degree of trust in one another, but so long as no one is at risk of being hurt, can be very enjoyable. If you are not very inventive yourself, you may like to look at books like Nancy Friday's *My Secret Garden*, which is a collection of women's sexual fantasies.

Talking it over

Whatever your particular sexual difficulty, it is vital to talk it over and try to pinpoint the underlying reasons. You may feel that none of the suggestions in the previous pages applies to you, and yet there may still be a lack of response on one side or the other which needs to be resolved.

It may be that the whole relationship is in difficulty (see p.46). It may be that one of you has suffered a recent bereavement: such loss can lead to a complete sexual 'freezing' which it can be hard for either partner to understand. When one partner has been ill, or suffers from heart trouble or high blood pressure, for example, the

Love-making positions

Physical and emotional problems may lead you to re-appraise your approach to love-making as a couple. These suggestions may help in some circumstances.

For whatever reason, a man in late middle-age may find himself temporarily impotent. It can help if his partner sits astride him so that she can gently guide his penis into position, even if it is not fully erect.

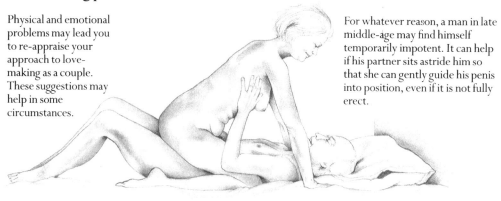

Allowing the man to enter from behind avoids pressure on the breasts or abdomen after a woman has had a mastectomy or hysterectomy. It is a comforting position emotionally as well.

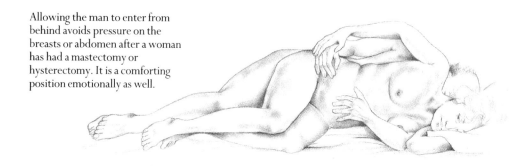

other is often frightened to make a sexual approach for fear of hurting or over-exerting him or her, while the 'patient' meanwhile may be feeling too rejected to make the first move.

Or it can be that one partner, most often the woman, never really enjoyed sex and is only too glad to use 'getting on' as an excuse to stop altogether. When only one partner feels this way, it is very sad, since as we have seen it is just at this period that sex can actually be better than ever before, when a couple can really concentrate on each other and may also most need one another. It is never too late to learn to enjoy sex: for a woman to become orgasmic and a man to learn to arouse and satisfy his partner, so if the relationship is good in other ways, a couple can derive much help from seeing a sex therapist. Sex is not just for the young, and nor is sex therapy.

Occasionally neither partner is strongly motivated to continue with their sex life. If both truly feel this way, and it is not just a reaction to feeling hurt or rejected, or because they have never learned to enjoy sex, then that is fine too. There is no law that says we all have to continue to be sexually active for ever. But for those who do continue their sexual relationship, there is great comfort, nurturing and delight to be had. As Browning said: 'Grow old along with me, The best is yet to be . . .'

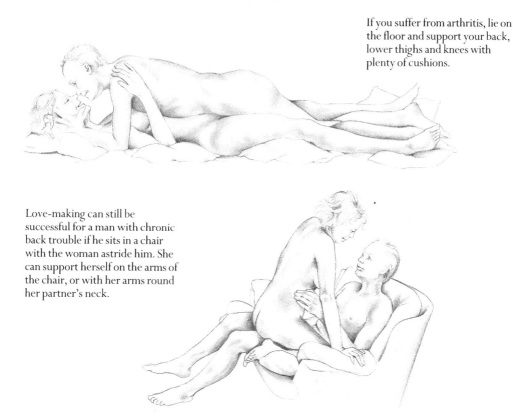

If you suffer from arthritis, lie on the floor and support your back, lower thighs and knees with plenty of cushions.

Love-making can still be successful for a man with chronic back trouble if he sits in a chair with the woman astride him. She can support herself on the arms of the chair, or with her arms round her partner's neck.

RELATIONSHIPS

Family changes

When children
leave home

It may well be true that 'the best is yet to be', but meanwhile all our relationships, and especially those with partner and family, have to undergo some quite substantial changes.

Couples who have been married for a long while and brought up children probably have to face the biggest change of all: from one day to the next it seems, the house has turned from being the neighbourhood coffee bar, football stadium, beauty parlour, recording studio or computer laboratory into an empty, echoing shell. And however much you may have been looking forward to this moment, it can still be quite a shock when it comes.

Women tend to feel the difference more painfully than men, and it is not unusual for a woman to go through a period of depression when the last child leaves home (although of course this may in part be due to the hormonal changes that are often taking place at the same time). I remember feeling like the walking wounded for weeks, and one woman put it even more graphically: 'When the tide of my children's needs had suddenly receded, I felt like a beached whale, gasping for air.'

This can be a delicate moment for a couple. Suddenly the whole focus is on their own relationship, which may not have been central for twenty years or more. Can the relationship stand it? Does it indeed still exist, or did it slip away unnoticed while life revolved around the children? 'What do we talk about when we don't talk about the children?' wailed one wife, confused and distressed despite being happily married, 'and how do I shop or cook for just two people?' The husband meanwhile may be feeling hurt that he is no longer enough for his wife; that just when he was looking forward to a bit of peace and quiet and the two of them being on their own, she is in mourning for the hurly-burly. No wonder this is a peak period for marriage break-ups. When children have been the cement that have kept a couple together, their leaving can expose

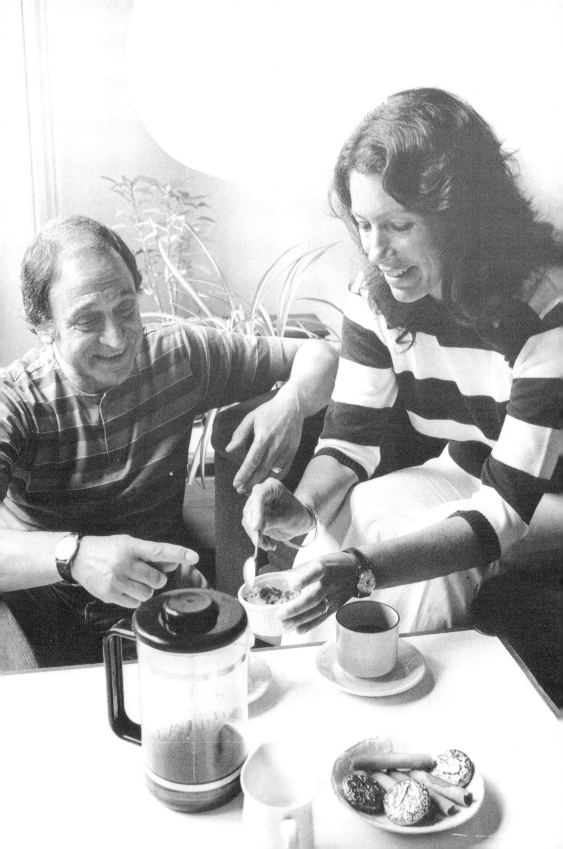

the arid cracks that have grown between them.

Moreover, watching the young take flight can make being grounded in mid-life painful to accept, and it is hard not to envy them their youth, their unlimited future, their freedom and their sexuality. A 'last fling' affair, especially with a younger partner, is one path that both men and women sometimes take to grab back a little of that youth, to dissociate themselves from their partner's 'middle agedness', and to reassure themselves that they are still alive and attractive. Such affairs can only too easily precipitate the break-up of the marriage (see p.42), but where there is enough good will and understanding between husband and wife, they can also lead to a new beginning in the relationship.

The childless couple   When a couple have not had children, whether by choice or not, there may be a critical period of regret as the woman approaches the menopause. She may for a while feel utterly consumed by what she has missed; men too can feel it quite as acutely as women. 'I feel eaten up with the longing to have had children,' one man said, as the couple tried to come to terms with the fact that now they never would. This takes great sensitivity on both sides, and it is especially important not to apportion blame, but rather to acknowledge and share the sense of loss.

The late pregnancy   Some women of course do have children in their 40s, sometimes the first, or perhaps because of a second marriage, the first for a long time. Either way, this can lead to immense changes in their lives, with psychological, social and economic adjustments to be made.

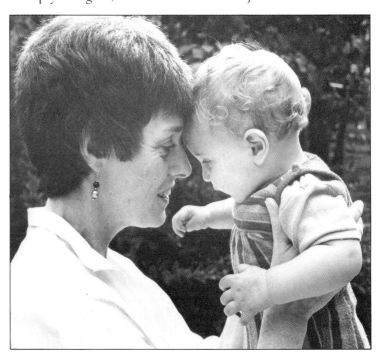

Late babies can give special delight, and an older mother is often better able to give herself whole-heartedly to the experience of having children.

There are advantages in having a baby at this age, despite the slightly greater physical risks involved. The baby, unless conceived by mistake during the menopause (and often even then), will almost certainly be a much desired one, and the mother's greater maturity and confidence may allow her to enjoy the child more whole-heartedly than younger women sometimes do.

Such babies usually give great delight, but there may be some surprising, sometimes quite hurtful, reactions from outsiders, and even from the woman's own family. Teenage and older children may be thrilled at the prospect of a new baby in the family, but their reactions can also prove disappointing. They may be embarrassed, 'disgusted' even, at their mother's pregnancy, which can stir up all kinds of unresolved feelings of sibling rivalry and about their own sexuality. Where step-children are concerned, the situation can be particularly delicate.

However hurtful such reactions may be, a mother will need to deal with them together with her partner (perhaps with the help of professional counselling), so that they do not become destructive to the family.

Re-discovering your partner

As a couple grow older they usually have more time to spend together, with less distraction from children or careers. A marriage can sometimes go on to 'automatic pilot' for years while family and job seem to demand all the attention and energy, so this can be a tricky but rewarding time of re-discovery. And 're-discovering' includes allowing the other to have changed. We often expect our nearest and dearest to remain just as they always were, and it is tempting to continue to relate to them as though this were so. Marriages that are based on such automatic responses are dead at the heart: only by really listening to the other, accepting the changes that maturity has brought, sharing one's thoughts and allowing for the other's concerns, can the marriage continue to live and flourish.

Accepting the aging process

It is also important, and not always easy, to allow the other to age. Watching one's partner go grey or bald, seeing him or her go slowly up the stairs instead of bounding up two steps at a time, needing more rest or getting a little hard of hearing, can be difficult to accept because it brings us up with a jolt against our own aging. It is easier to be irritated with the other than to recognize that we too are not as young as we may still like to think of ourselves.

Making room for each other

When a husband retires the wife sometimes has an added problem in making room for him in the house, which may have been her exclusive daytime domain for decades. 'He is under my feet all day' is a common grumble, which takes little account of the husband's own struggle to find a new role and new occupations for himself. And one wife, fully sympathetic to what her husband was going through, nonetheless said, 'I feel as though he is watching me all the time, so I feel guilty if I have a rest or sit down to read a book during the day, or have a long chat on the phone with a friend. If I'm not busy all the time I'm afraid he'll think I have just been slacking all these years.'

The best way to resolve this, as most other problems in marriage, is to talk openly about how both of you feel, and to find a way of accommodating each partner's needs. Marriages do not remain static any more than individuals do, and have to be re-negotiated, tacitly or explicitly, at various stages. When children leave home and when one or both partners retire from work are only two such moments in a series of critical transitions. There is always a choice at such times: a couple can refuse to acknowledge that anything is altered but each nurse their own grievances, or they can accept that the needs of each have changed, but so too have the opportunities for both.

Making a new start

Sometimes quite simple things, like rearranging or redecorating the home, are symbolic of this being the beginning of a new phase, and often couples move house at this point, not just for economic reasons, but because the old one has become a museum to a life that is now past. And it is necessary, though not always easy, to let it go.

Money is often a little less tight once the children are independent, so this can be a time for finding new occupations and interests, both ones that can be shared and ones that each can pursue on his or her own. A network of friends, both joint and individual, also becomes more important if a couple is not to become isolated and totally interdependent.

Though some couples like to do everything together, most feel the need for space for each individual if they and the partnership are to continue to grow and flourish: not since Adam and Eve have husband and wife actually been joined at the rib. One of the best recipes for marriage, which applies as much or more to maturity as to the beginning of marriage, is in Kahlil Gibran's poem:

Love one another but make not a bond of love:
Let it rather be a moving sea between the shores of your souls.
Fill each other's cup, but drink not from one cup.
Give one another of your bread, but eat not from the same
loaf.
Sing and dance together and be joyous, but let each one of
you be alone,
Even as the strings of a lute are alone though they quiver
with the same music.

The single woman

Not all women of course have a husband or a partner at this stage. Some have never married and may be perfectly happy to continue to live their lives on their own; others fling themselves into a frenzied search for a partner 'before it's too late', or they resign themselves to never marrying. Yet they may still marry, and some late marriages bring great happiness, but on the whole statistics are against this happening for many women in this age group.

Divorce and widowhood

Women who face divorce or widowhood during this period have quite different adjustments to make. In different ways, both have to go through a period of mourning, with all its stages of grief, rage and guilt, before they feel whole again. Guilt, however irrational, seems to be an abiding theme, whether it is guilt at the failure of the marriage, or guilt at having 'allowed' the other to die, and it can take a long time to overcome this.

Changes to social life

Most women find that the pattern of their lives changes drastically once they are on their own. Social life is still largely built on the Noah's Ark principle of 'two-by-two', and a woman alone can have a hard time. Most find that their network of contacts changes, and their social life revolves more around other women than before. Widows especially may feel themselves to be very isolated, since death is still to some extent a taboo subject. Only too often neighbours and acquaintances shun the recently bereaved – 'They even cross the road to avoid having to speak to me' one recently bereaved woman found.

When the death of a partner is sudden, as can happen frequently given the high incidence of heart disease in western society, the surviving partner can be in shock long after she or anyone else will probably realize. But whether the death comes suddenly or after a long illness, a widow needs both time and space for herself to give herself up freely to her grief, and also the loving help and support of friends and family. Such women will also need to rely more than they have ever done on the help of professionals, like bank managers, solicitors or doctors, and when the first period of mourning is over, it is important not only to accept help, but also to reach out for it – people often hesitate to offer for fear of intruding.

Children and grandchildren

Our relationships with our children undergo the most crucial changes at this time. If the children are still in their adolescence while their mother is going through the menopause, she may find their turmoil and struggles particularly hard to tolerate, since they so nearly resemble her own. As children grow into adulthood and independence, their need to separate from their parents may come just at the moment when the parents, and especially a mother who is on her own, may be feeling particularly vulnerable and dependent on them for companionship, friendship, love and support. However hard, letting them go is vital, and it must be with your full support and approval, so that they do not feel burdened with guilt at leaving.

Letting go of guilt

It is time too to let go of our own guilt towards our children. Everyone thinks they have done something wrong in their children's upbringing, yet we all probably did the best we could at the time, and whatever difficulties the children may now have in their own lives and relationships can no longer be our fault. Most of us are so conditioned to feeling responsible for our children's development that it is hard to stop feeling guilty. No doubt if we had our time over again we would do it better, but once they are grown up they must take responsibility for themselves and for their actions and interactions.

Accepting your children's relationships

This becomes particularly relevant when they start bringing back boyfriends and girlfriends. Classically this is harder for fathers to bear, who may feel, even if unacknowledged, envy of their sons or possessive about their daughters. But mothers too have to let go of some of the intimacy they may have had with both daughters and sons, who will no longer be so ready to confide in them. And it can be hard too to tolerate the friends we do not like, though we have to remember that only a few young people are lucky enough to recognize what is right for them before they have experienced what is wrong.

The relationship with a daughter growing into womanhood can be especially rewarding at this time.

One of the hardest moments for a parent is to watch a child making a serious mistake in choosing a partner. Being the parent of adults is to feel responsibility without having power (though we

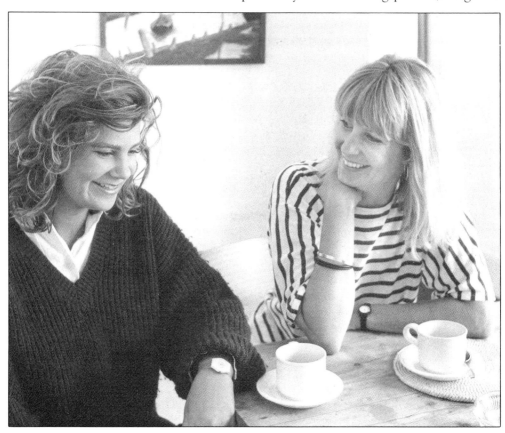

may still have influence), and we have to learn to accept this.

When children marry

When eventually the children marry, 'letting go' becomes even more crucial, and we have to find the delicate balance between accepting that the child's centre of gravity now finally lies outside the original family circle and at the same time welcoming the new member into the family.

The birth of grandchildren

When grandchildren arrive a balance has to be found again, this time between being available without being intrusive or over-bearing. There is another adjustment to come to terms with: suddenly your own children no longer see you as their parents, but as their children's grandparents – which is a whole new identity. This can be particularly hard for women who have grandchildren while they themselves are still relatively young (perhaps even having a late baby of their own at the same time). They may be quite unready to accept the traditional 'grandmother' role, and in reject-ing the role, may be at risk of seeming to reject the child. Unless everyone concerned is able to explain and express their feelings, this can be a confusing situation, especially for the young children concerned. But on the whole, most people find that grandchildren are a pleasure – so much love without responsibility!

Grandchildren can give unalloyed pleasure – so much love without responsibility.

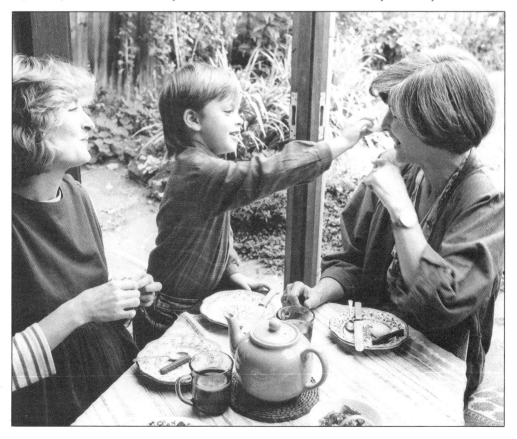

As parents age

All this time we may be not only wives, mothers and possibly grandmothers, but also daughters. If our parents are still alive they will be elderly and may need a lot of attention and nurturing. This reversal of roles can be hard to accept: we do not expect to parent our parents, and yet may have years ahead when it will be necessary. When parents become dependent, it is especially difficult if the relationship has not been an easy one in the past, for it is necessary to give up the old resentments and quarrels.

Caring for an elderly parent

Yet again a difficult balance has to be struck between taking care of an elderly parent and not sacrificing your own life or family to them. Women who do not devote themselves totally to the care of an elderly parent are often obsessed with guilt (that dangerous hallmark of women in mid-life). Even when parents do not become wholly dependent, they can still claim a large amount of attention at this time. Watching my own mother struggle with gallant independence through a difficult old age, I realized that I was in danger of becoming on one hand so obsessed with guilt towards her, and on the other dreading old age for myself, that I was at risk of failing to live and enjoy my life *now*. Some women find their lives dominated by the need to look after an elderly parent. Our society has not found a solution to the problems of the increasingly ageing population, but giving up one life for another cannot be the answer.

Bereavement

When parents die, and especially the parent of one's own sex, we become the frontier generation. However old they were and however timely their death may be, you have to go through a period of mourning before you can come to terms with the loss, and that bereavement, however much you must have expected it, can for a time rock relationships, especially that with your partner. Women frequently find that they cannot enjoy sex for a while after a parent has died (see p.44), while some take refuge from grief in almost frenzied sexual activity. Either way can put strains on a partnership, and needs sensitive understanding on both sides.

Relationships at work

Attitudes to work may well change too at this time. Some women start a completely new work pattern: the successful career woman may decide the time has come to give up the career and to develop her artistic talents; the women who has always worked for the community may decide to try her hand at starting a business; the housewife who has hitherto devoted herself to looking after the home and family may decide it is time to take a degree or to look for a job.

Changing direction

Not that it is easy for women to start a new job or career in mid-life, but there are organizations designed to help, such as 'New Directions' in Britain, which runs workshops to help women find in which direction their talents lie, and in America a group of older women have founded OWL (Older Women's League), a pressure group to fight for the rights of older women. 'Don't Agonize,

Organize' is their slogan, and perhaps it is time we banded together in Britain to fight the same good fight. (See also p.124).

Of course not every woman wants to start a new job or career. Those who have always worked outside the home may simply enjoy the fact that now they can concentrate on their careers without feeling torn between the demands of the job and those of the family. Many women justly feel that the time has come at last when they can work less hard, relax more, enjoy their leisure quietly, and above all without the guilt of feeling that they should be doing something else. This can also be the time to allow yourself to expend less energy, to live less hectically and to spend more time by yourself and for yourself.

Being yourself

Ultimately, the most important relationship any of us will ever have is with ourselves. Yet as women we have long been accustomed to defining ourselves through our relationships with others. We are somebody's wife, perhaps somebody's mistress, someone's mother, often also someone's daughter or sister. Many of us, if asked to describe ourselves, would find it hard not to do so in terms of the other people in our lives. (Try it!)

As we get older, this becomes more difficult. Many of the old roles no longer apply (it feels foolish to introduce yourself as the mother of four children when those children's ages range from 20 to 30!) and we may not yet know how to replace them. This period is one of reassessment, a time to rediscover and redefine ourselves, to find strengths that have perhaps been dormant, or to use old skills in new ways. As in adolescence, there can be a period of agonizing confusion and even despair that we will ever find a way forward again. But, just as in adolescence, there is also the excitement of new opportunities and new challenges ahead. As Susan Sontag wrote in her essay on 'The Double Standard of Aging': 'Women have another option. They can aspire to be wise, not merely nice; to be competent, not merely helpful; to be strong, not merely graceful; to be ambitious for themselves, not merely for themselves in relation to men and children.'

Seeing oneself directly, and not through the lens of others, can be very liberating. The women's movement has fought hard for all women to be treated as full human beings, and this is the time to take responsibility for ourselves. No longer can we hide behind our old roles; no longer can we plead other people's needs of us as an excuse for allowing ourselves to remain underdeveloped. Even if we have never done so before, we have finally now to take a realistic assessment of ourselves, to recognize our individual strengths and weaknesses, to acknowledge that we are the person we have become and can no longer blame our parents, our upbringing or our present circumstances for everything we do nor what we leave undone. The choices are ours and from now on, 'the buck stops here'.

TAKING CARE OF
YOURSELF

Looking your best

Most of us, I am sure, always intended to age gracefully, but that was in the days when we were convinced that wrinkles, crepey necks, blue veins on the legs and double chins were never going to happen to *us*. Once we reach the stage where signs of aging begin to appear, we find them rather harder to accept. Yet accept them we must.

Looking (and acting) our age is a delicate matter, since, in so far as there are any norms, they are constantly changing. Most of us probably look younger at 40 and at 50 than our mothers did at that age (better nutrition and health care, changing life-styles, fashion and advances in cosmetics are all in our favour), but however much we may pride ourselves that we look younger than our age, we cannot deny that we looked younger twenty or even ten years ago than we do now.

That does not mean to say that we cannot and should not look good, not 'for our age' (that insulting parenthesis) but *at* our age. Women can be beautiful at 40 as they can at 20, and they can still be beautiful when they are 80 or 90. It is a different beauty, one that owes as much to personality, experience and attitudes as to bone structure and skin quality. It is important to recognize this, so that we do not grieve over every new grey hair or wrinkle. A Dorian Grey face that remains totally unlined would be eerily disconcerting; faces that express a personality, that have been 'lived in', are far more attractive than a bland and lacquered beautician's mask.

Feeling good

How we see and present ourselves is intimately linked with how we feel about ourselves. If we subscribe to the general conspiracy that aging men can continue to be attractive but aging women cannot, then growing older will be a depressing experience, and we will either let our appearance go completely, or frenziedly try to preserve body and face with all the artifice we can afford. But if we can accept that being, and looking, the age we are is no disgrace, if

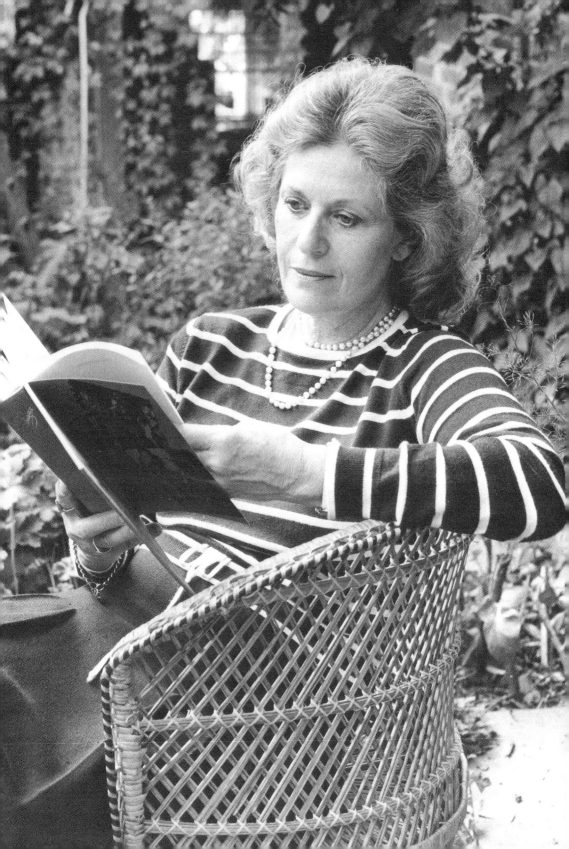

we can allow ourselves and our faces to tell the truth, then we will not have damaged our self-respect, and we can still look our best.

Accepting the fact of aging is not the same as letting our general health, and with it our appearance, go rapidly downhill. Both need care and attention, and rather more so now than when we were younger. And both are closely interlinked. It is a benign circle; the better we feel, the better we look, and vice versa.

Keeping fit

Keeping fit, therefore, is the obvious and vital prerequisite for good health and the good looks that health can bring. When we are young, most of us are lucky enough to take health for granted, but as we get older we need to work at it if we are to preserve our energies, vitality and zest. The second section of this book is devoted to explaining and describing the kind of exercises that will keep our skin, muscles, bones and joints in good shape (see p.64). But that is not the whole story. What we eat and drink also plays a large part in keeping our bodies functioning at their best.

Diet and weight

We in the West are over-obsessed with weight but it is true that being overweight is bad for your health. Too thin can be almost as bad as too fat, and some women have to work hard to maintain their proper body weight (see p.22). But the plain fact is that as we get older the metabolic rate slows down; we simply need fewer calories for the amount of energy we are expending. To misquote the Red Queen, we just have to eat less to stay in the same place. Sad but true, and especially sad for those for whom eating and drinking remain one of life's special pleasures. Yet no one would suggest that we should give up enjoying food, or even alcohol in moderation, except when there are special medical reasons. We just need to eat

This chart shows average weights, according to the size of your frame.

height without shoes	small frame	medium frame	large frame	height without shoes	small frame	medium frame	large frame
cm	kg	kg	kg	ft in	lb	lb	lb
142	39	44	48	4 8	87	97	106
145	40	45	50	4 9	89	99	109
147	42	46	51	4 10	92	102	112
150	43	48	53	4 11	95	105	116
152	44	49	54	5 0	97	108	119
155	45	50	55	5 1	100	111	122
157	47	52	57	5 2	103	115	126
160	48	54	59	5 3	106	118	130
162	50	56	62	5 4	110	123	135
165	51	58	63	5 5	114	127	139
167	53	60	65	5 6	117	131	144
170	56	62	67	5 7	121	135	148
172	57	63	69	5 8	125	139	152
175	58	65	71	5 9	128	143	157
177	60	67	73	5 10	132	147	161

and drink less, and more sensibly.

Eating sensibly

Fat or thin, or even if we have the ideal weight, eating the right kinds of food and avoiding the wrong ones is a vital part of maintaining health. This is especially important for anyone living on their own: they may feel it is not worth shopping or cooking for one, and the temptation can be great to reach for convenience foods, most of which contain harmful additives.

The picture of what constitutes sensible eating can be quite confusing, as every year we are told of some new item of food that is bad for us. One year we are all adjured to switch to margarine and polyunsaturated fats only, the next it is 'welcome back to butter', to give just one example. Nonetheless, a few facts emerge clearly.

Some facts about food

1 Fewer calories mean less weight gain. It has been estimated that whereas it takes about 15 calories a day to maintain one pound of body weight, you need to cut out 3500 calories to *lose* one pound. But counting calories is a deadly game which no one should play for too long. For the long term it is much better to acquaint yourself with the relative calorific values of the basic foods, and then to keep a balance in your daily intake. And that does not mean denying yourself the occasional treat – just compensate for it the next day.

2 Remaining active and taking plenty of exercise (see p.67), together with sensible eating, should maintain most women at a steady weight. If you have a lot of weight to lose, then you will need to take much more care with your diet and probably step up the amount of exercise, but crash or fad diets, although they may seem to have startling results to begin with, rarely do any long-term good. Usually it is chiefly excess fluid that is actually lost, so that as soon as a normal diet is resumed, the weight very quickly comes back. Moreover, though it may be all right for a young girl to lose weight rapidly, it is rarely flattering for older women to do so; generally we seem to lose it in our faces first, so that we begin to look haggard or sagging, rather than lean and fit. Much better to lose slowly over a period of time while exercising regularly, so that the facial and other muscles can remain taut, and the weight loss is permanent and not just to be regained the moment we return to normal eating.

3 Fats, especially the saturated variety (ie those derived from animals and animal products), should be consumed in moderation only. Not only do they contribute to weight gain, but they are also associated with heart disease.

4 Salt (sodium) can exacerbate high blood pressure, to which older women are in any case prone (see p.23). It increases water retention (hence weight gain) and can aggravate the bloating from which some women suffer, particularly during the menopause. Remember that salt is not only present when you add it to your food, but has already been added to many processed foods.

5 Sugar, especially refined sugar, is also a potential health hazard. It

is likely to increase the risk of heart disease, and our bodies process it more slowly as we get older. Sugar has to be cut out of your diet anyway if you become diabetic (see p.24), so it is worth remembering that even savoury processed foods often have sugar added to increase the flavour.

6 Vitamins are vital, all of them: Vitamin A, the B complex, C and E, and also calcium (see p.22). Acquaint yourself with the vitamin constituents of everyday foods, and try to have some of each in fresh fruit and vegetables every day. You may also like to take vitamin supplements, especially if you do not have access to really fresh fruit and vegetables.

7 Water is wonderful. Good water, purified if necessary, contains vitamins and minerals, and is also calorie-free. It helps to keep the skin supple and moisturized. You should drink several glasses (some say eight!) every day.

8 Finally, it is no news that smoking is bad for you. But the risks are not only of lung cancer. Smoking restricts the blood vessels and can lead to heart disease; it can affect the calcium balance of the body, increasing the risk of osteoporosis (see p.20); it wars with the body's uptake of vitamins and it can affect the skin, possibly causing increased wrinkling. Give it up if you possibly can!

Getting rest

Our sleep patterns change as we get older. Most people find they need less sleep at night, while a short nap in the afternoon, given the opportunity, can be a great energy restorer. If you can accept that you need less sleep and can use the waking hours to read or listen to music without disturbing anyone, or just to think constructively about any problems, you will not feel the time has been wasted.

Unfortunately many people find that dwelling on their problems at night makes them more wakeful and tense. They then begin to worry that they will never get to sleep, which in turn increases the tension and sleeplessness. Getting through those bleak hours before dawn, when the metabolism and therefore the morale are at their lowest, can be a struggle. Many women suffer from some degree of depression during these night hours, and for many it is a time to mull over the negative aspects of their lives, and especially to indulge in that favourite pastime, guilt. A positive effort to turn black thoughts into pleasant memories or day dreams, or to empty the mind and relax the body, can actually help not only to keep depression at bay but also to bring back sleep. Try to use the relaxation technique described on page 119; then even if you can't sleep, your body and mind will still feel refreshed.

Insomnia

Real insomnia, however, can be a warning signal that all is not well, and may be a symptom of illness or serious depression. It should not be ignored but should be checked by a doctor. It is possible that he or she may want to prescribe tranquillizers or sleeping pills in this situation. These are sometimes helpful at a particularly difficult moment when the mind is too distressed to allow the body the quiet and rest it needs, either to recover from a physical trauma or to cope with the challenge of a crisis situation. But they should be taken for short periods only – if at all. If your doctor does suggest them, discuss why and for how long he or she thinks you should take them. It is only too easy to become dependent on these drugs which offer no cure in themselves but only suppress the symptoms.

Coping with stress

The stress from which many people suffer at this period of their lives, either from pressure at work, from family demands or other life circumstances, can take its toll, especially as an all too common way of dealing with stress is to turn to alcohol, smoking or tranquillizers. Far better instead, when you feel the pressure mounting, to take some exercise (even a short run or walk can reduce tension remarkably, see p.67) or take just ten minutes off to practise relaxation (see p.119). Both refresh the spirit and renew the energies. Having a massage is another excellent way to reduce tension. It is a treat that is well worth giving yourself.

Care of the skin

We have only to look at the skin on the inside of our arms to realize that if the rest of us – especially our face – is no longer covered by soft, fine-textured, unblemished skin, it is exposure and lack of care as much as aging that are to blame. As we get older, the skin loses collagen (a natural protein) and so gets thinner and has to be handled with extra care – no pulling, stretching or scrubbing.

Dry skin

The sweat and oil glands that lubricate the skin also slow down, and most skin types, especially after the menopause and even if they are naturally oily, need extra moisture to prevent excessive drying. This does not need to be an expensive lotion, but it is a good idea to apply some moisturizer during the day whether you wear make-up or not. Most people apply moisturizer at night when it is actually least beneficial, since the skin will not absorb it nearly so well when the whole body is at rest. Better to use a moisturizing mask or even to invest in an occasional professional skin treatment.

Wrinkles

Though often associated with dry skin, wrinkles are actually the result of genetic changes, and the tendency towards wrinkles is largely inherited. However, a dry skin will show wrinkles more, and if you are prone to them, moisturizing is even more essential.

A sun tan also accentuates wrinkles, as well as being a health hazard. Attractive as a sun tan may be, we should avoid the sun, particularly on the face, as we get older, not only because of the risk of skin cancer but also because after the first glow of the tan has worn off, the effect is usually an unattractively aging one.

'Liver' spots

'Liver' or 'sun' spots (most frequently found on the back of the hands) have no connection with the liver and little with the sun, even though they look like giant freckles. They may in part be due to exposure, but are more likely the result of hormonal changes leading to a change of pigmentation, so the other common name, 'age spots', is, I am afraid, probably more accurate. If they bother you you can have them removed by a dermatologist who will freeze them with liquid nitrogen: don't try to deal with them yourself without having first consulted a doctor.

Sagging features

The subcutaneous fat which plumps out our faces shrinks naturally with age, leaving sagging lines around the eyes and eyelids and under the chin, as well as hollowing the cheeks. Though exercising the muscles around the jaw and neck (see p.76) can help to keep double chins at bay (and so does sleeping without a pillow) we cannot altogether prevent these signs of aging.

Cosmetic surgery

This raises the question of cosmetic surgery. And, if you can afford it, why not? If your double chin, your drooping eyelids or your sagging bust really depress you, you may like to investigate what cosmetic surgery could do for you. But shop around, see at least three different surgeons and do not necessarily go for the cheapest nor for the one who promises the most dramatic results. Rather, assess how realistic are the promises – ask previous patients if you can. If anything go for the surgeon who is most conservative in his claims – better to be agreeably surprised by the results than disappointed. And remember in any case that these are still only temporary, even if relatively long-term, improvements. Ultimately none of us can escape for ever from the process of aging.

Care of the teeth

Although teeth should not be a particular problem (the rate of dental decay generally slows down in our 40s and 50s), our gums become more vulnerable with age. They shrink a little – hence the term 'long in the tooth' – and they become more prone to infection. As gums shrink gaps between the teeth increase, requiring more attention to keep clean. Strict oral hygiene with dental floss and probe toothbrushes and regular visits to the dentist remain as important now as when we were children. And if teeth are lost, they should be replaced by a crown or bridge, for gaps left in the mouth can distort the bite and lead to further decay in the remaining teeth.

Looking after your hair

Hair also shows some changes. Although women are luckier than men in that we rarely go bald, the rate at which the hair grows and the hairs replace themselves slows down with age, so that some thinning generally occurs. And of course sooner or later almost all of us begin to have grey hairs – which simply means that the new hairs that grow have little or no pigmentation.

Deciding to dye

To dye or not to dye is a question most women will ask themselves at some stage, and will answer according to temperament, self-image and how grey or white hair actually suits them. The only general rule must be that if it is to be, then t'were better it were done well, preferably professionally, and it must be done frequently. Nothing is more aging than white roots showing on the scalp of a raven or red-head, and colouring that is crudely or unevenly applied almost always shows up, especially in sunlight. Harsh colour can also make a face look more faded and lined. Highlights or sun streaks in the hair, on the other hand, can be very attractive and give a lift to an otherwise dull or lifeless head of hair.

The case for good grooming

Good grooming and a sense of her own style are a mature woman's best allies. A 'sweet disorder of the dress' may look enchanting on a young girl, but an older woman will probably just look sloppy. That is not to say that we have to be dressed up all the time or that our clothes should be middle-aged: jeans and T-shirts *can* look as good on an older woman as on a teenager, but whereas almost all teenagers will look good in them, all mature women do not.

Knowing your style, recognizing what looks good on you and what doesn't, making a realistic assessment of yourself and dressing to suit you *now*, not as you used to look nor as you hope to look when you have lost a few pounds; using make-up that is fashionable now, not that was in vogue a quarter of a century ago, and using it in a way that enhances the face you have now, not the one you had when you were a young girl; wearing a hairstyle that flatters you and suits your hair, and not the style you have always worn, or that your hair used to fall into naturally, even though it won't quite behave in the way it used to do; all these are stratagems for looking – and feeling – confident and alive.

The best of maturity

We have a lot on our side at this time. Hair-styles are soft and natural, and there are perms and lotions that will keep the hair in shape and give it body without having to wear the corrugated iron waves we used to associate with the middle-aged. Make-up has become so varied and so subtle that with a little skill and perhaps some professional help we can learn to highlight our better points and draw attention away from some of the signs of aging. And above all fashion has probably never been so liberated. Anything goes, and nothing is considered to be more suitable for one age group than another. Any woman at any age now can find clothes in almost any price range that are comfortable as well as flattering and that she can enjoy wearing.

And enjoyment is the key word. This is the time to indulge ourselves, to cherish and even pamper ourselves. A massage, a facial, a manicure or a pedicure, whatever we can afford to do that will raise our morale and make us feel good about ourselves is time and money well spent. Just as we should have regular breast examinations, cervical smears and blood pressure tests, so we need to take regular stock of our appearance and occasionally treat ourselves to some small luxury. Now is the time to think of ourselves, and even occasionally, and with a good conscience, to put ourselves first.

EXERCISES FOR FITNESS & HEALTH

Why exercise?

Few people can have failed to notice the tremendous emphasis on 'fitness' these days. Newspapers, television, magazines and books are all filled with exercise programmes, every one different, every one claiming to be the best! It may leave you feeling rather confused, and if you have not taken much exercise for some time you may be put off before you start! Perhaps you feel that because you are older it is too late to do anything about your body and its shortcomings. However, exercising is not only about improving and maintaining good health, but also preventing and alleviating problems that can arise at this time of life, and later on.

Have you noticed that your legs ache and you get a bit more out of breath going up stairs; that your shoulder joints feel a little stiff when you are putting on a jacket or coat; that your neck doesn't turn as easily as it used to when you are backing the car? These are all small limitations which gradually creep up on us over the years but which can be improved with regular exercise. Feeling and looking fit and well in your forties and fifties increases self-confidence and enables you to keep up with younger friends, children and even grandchildren, and most importantly gives you a positive approach to the years ahead.

What is fitness?

So what do we mean by 'fitness'? It is a combination of flexibility, strength, stamina and endurance, co-ordination and balance, and last but not least, the ability to relax. Feeling fit means being able to do what you want to do, when you want to do it.

Flexibility

Flexibility is the ability to move the muscles and joints through their full range. As we grow older, flexibility is one of the first things to go, often through lack of regular physical activity. Almost every movement of the body involves the shortening and contracting of muscles; these actions repeated over and over again can build up into tension and tightening which leave the body feeling stiff and

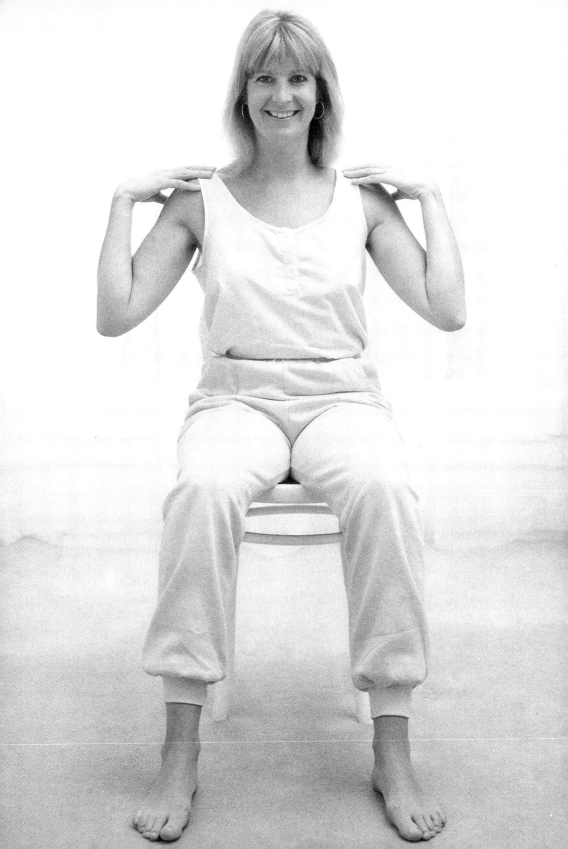

impede good circulation. Tight muscles also hamper the joints, preventing their full range of movement. This forces the body constantly to be working against itself – more energy is needed for each activity, building up to increased fatigue.

Stretching exercises are among the most useful for improving flexibility. Stretching lengthens the muscles, releases the tightness around the joints and allows blood to circulate freely. Some good slow stretching exercises performed regularly will keep your body lithe and young-looking, and release energy into the body.

Strength

The skeleton forms the framework of the body and it needs to be fully supported in order to function properly. The weaker the supporting muscles are, the more effort is involved in performing even the simplest movements. Sitting up straight, walking up stairs, running for the bus, carrying a heavy shopping bag or taking out the garbage – all these every day tasks become harder to do. It is therefore important to exercise regularly to strengthen and maintain the muscles throughout the body, so try to work on this programme at least three times a week.

Stamina and endurance

Another word for stamina is endurance – the ability to resist and recover from fatigue. As we grow older our reserves of physical energy drop – it takes longer to recover from a late night, an unexpected work load, illness and mental strain. Build up your stamina gradually, starting with the basic exercises and working towards a more vigorous activity to increase the capacity and efficiency of your heart and lungs and work your muscles harder.

Balance and co-ordination

Balance is an essential part of health. Being confident about your sense of balance will give you the ability to move about freely, especially as you grow older. Good posture is really a balancing act, so improved posture will lead to better balance in the body.

Relaxation

Relaxation is something which does not come easily to everyone. Some people feel they do not need it, saying, 'I sleep very well, so why should I need relaxation?' or 'I haven't got time for it', which so often means 'I don't want to make time'. But relaxation is very different from sleep. It is not only useful for a few minutes each day to help restore energy and give renewed vigour to carry on activities, it can also help to change one's attitude to the stresses and irritations of everyday life (see page 118).

Getting into shape

The exercises which follow will combine to help you improve on all the points described in the definition of fitness. Do not be discouraged if you are just starting to exercise after a long break of little or no physical activity. If you find it difficult to discipline yourself to exercise regularly, why not join forces with a friend or your partner; you will both benefit.

To begin with you may find that you perform better in one area than another, so work harder on your weaker points and notice the improvements. Aim for balance in the body so that you no longer favour one side more than the other. Become aware of the way in which you use your body in everyday life, and work towards eliminating the bad habits. The increased mobility and flexibility which come from regular exercise will encourage you to continue.

The need for exercise

Recent research has shown that regular physical activity can do a great deal to relieve anxiety and depression. In fact these conditions often accompany an inactive life-style; as the body is designed to be mobile, lack of adequate movement makes the whole system sluggish. Anxiety and depression often lead to sleeplessness, with a concomitant reliance on pills to induce sleep, plus increased smoking, consumption of alcohol and excessive eating, as well as other physical and mental problems. Taking up exercise of some sort, even if it is only a brisk walk to begin with, will have an invigorating effect on the body and help to relieve the lethargy often induced by anxiety or boredom, helping you to break out of the vicious circle of sleeplessness and pills, and moving you instead into a positive state of mental and physical relaxation.

Combining the exercises with sport

You may already have been exercising for some time or take part in some regular sport, in which case you may feel that the exercises that follow are too easy or slow for you. Don't be fooled however: most of us benefit from more general exercises. If you play a regular game of squash or tennis for example, your arm, shoulder and leg muscles may well be strong, but how flexible are you? Have you checked your posture lately, have you noticed any reduction in the size of your waist and hips? It is not enough to have some strong muscles. Overall strength avoids overstraining those stronger muscles, and it is important to work on stretching them and on improving the flexibility of the joints.

If you use these exercises in conjunction with your regular sport, you will soon notice the benefits of working your body as a whole, rather than concentrating on one or two specific areas.

Check your health

A word of warning before you start on any exercise programme. If you have not taken up any exercise before, are in any doubt about your health, suffer from heart or respiratory problems, or are recovering from any illness or surgery, do check with your doctor first. It is quick and easy for your doctor to check your blood pressure and assure you that you will not be straining your body unduly. If you suffer from rheumatism or arthritis do not exercise when in pain or when taking pain-killers. Pain is always the body's warning sign, so be sensible and 'listen' to your body. The exercises given in this book should be suitable for everyone, but do not be in a hurry to attempt the more advanced ones (indicated where you see a suggested 'Progression'), before mastering the basic exercises. Above all enjoy yourself!

BASIC SKILLS: *POSTURE*

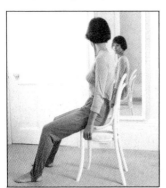

head straight
neck lengthened
shoulders down
ribs lifted
spine lengthened

pelvis centred

knees straight
but not braced

feet
hip-width apart

Correct posture

The most important sets of muscles involved in posture are the back muscles (working in conjunction with the abdominals), so they need to be strong and flexible (see p. 90). Weak back muscles tire easily and this leads to general slumping in the body (see p. 101). The importance of correct posture cannot be too strongly emphasised. As we grow older we cannot avoid the general deterioration of the discs between the vertebrae (the backbone), or the vertebrae themselves, the knee and hip joints, but the situation is going to be greatly worsened by poor posture which may compress and distort the discs unnecessarily and put strain on the joints.

Before starting any exercise routine, first check your posture. If you practise correcting it often, you will soon notice the difference in yourself – you will feel lighter, with more energy and vitality. By learning to lift your ribs away from your hips you expand the abdominal cavity, allowing for better breathing and uncramped internal organs.

Correct sitting posture

Exercise Sit sideways on to a large mirror, using a firm stool or straight-backed chair. Turn your head to watch yourself in the mirror. Keep your legs straight in front of you, hip-width apart, feet flat on the floor and slightly forward, and toes relaxed.

Centreing your pelvis Gently roll the top of the pelvis back so that you are sitting on the fleshy part of your buttocks, then roll it up and forwards. Repeat this movement backwards and forwards several times.

Centre your pelvis, feeling your sitting bones firmly underneath you. (Feel for these bones with your fingers if you are not sure where they

are.) Let your arms hang loosely by your sides, shoulders well down and back.

Lengthening your spine Now face forward and think about balancing your head, upper and lower torso one on top of the other over the pelvis. In this way the muscles work without undue strain. Breath in gently, and, as you breath out, lift and lengthen your body upwards, rather like a puppet on a string.

This lifting and lengthening of the body is the position to aim for throughout your daily life. It will soon become quite natural to you as your muscles strengthen and you become more aware of your body.

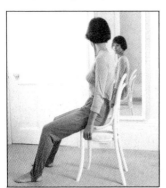
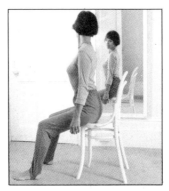
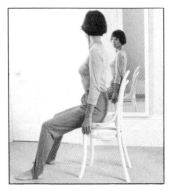

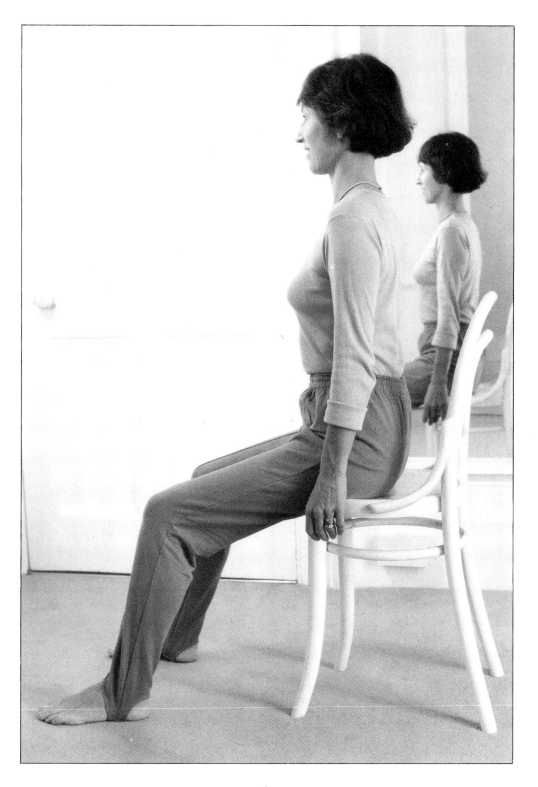

Correct standing posture

Distributing your weight
Stand at right angles to a full-length mirror with your feet hip-width apart and parallel. Watch yourself as you start by rocking gently backwards and forwards from the balls of the feet to the heels, then stand firmly distributing the weight evenly. Push your weight slightly towards the outside of the feet and relax your toes. Make sure that your feet are not rolling in, as this will put strain on the knees.

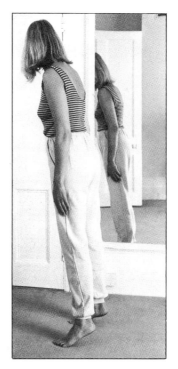 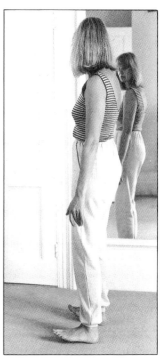

Centreing your pelvis Bend your knees slightly and rock your pelvis forwards and backwards gently a few times, then centre it and straighten your knees, without bracing them. Make sure that you have not clenched your buttocks.

Pull your shoulders down away from your ears and lengthen the back of the neck. Let your arms hang loosely by your sides. Imagine a straight line drawn from behind the ear, through the tip of the shoulder down your arm to just behind the ankle bone.

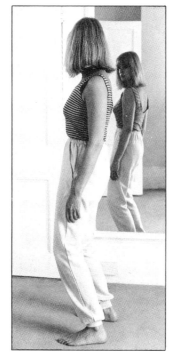 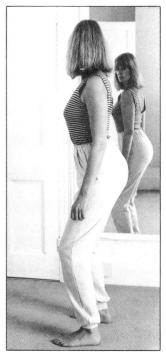

Lengthening your spine

Turn to face forwards. Breath in gently, and as you breath out lift your ribs away from your hips, lengthen your spine and feel your whole body lengthen upwards. Stand for a few minutes in this position, breathing well. Then start to move slowly but smoothly around the room without allowing your shoulders to stiffen, concentrating on your new posture as you do so.

With regular practice you will soon be able to feel when your posture is correct. Try this test for yourself – put on your favourite outfit and stand in front of the mirror, first in your habitual stance and then with correct posture; notice the difference. You will not be the only one to do so!

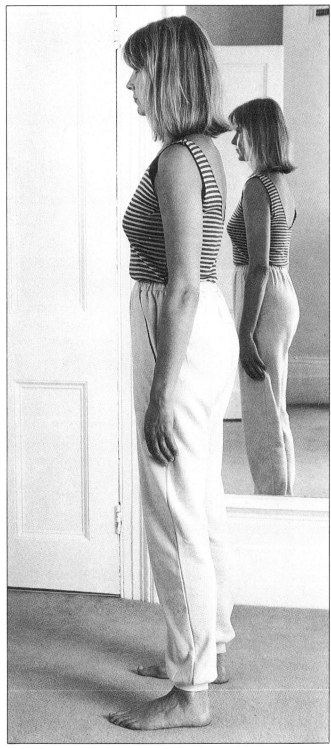

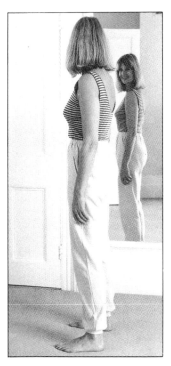

BREATHING

When we breathe, the diaphragm, the 'breathing muscle' which lies beneath the ribs, works with the intercostal muscles between the ribs to aid the action of the lungs. As we breathe *in*, the diaphragm moves down and the increased internal pressure forces the abdomen out. When we breathe *out*, the diaphragm rises and the abdomen flattens as the pressure is released, producing a natural massaging effect on the internal organs.

The process of growing older and lack of regular physical activity both lessen the elasticity of the lungs and the flexibility of the ribs. Regular exercise combined with good breathing will maintain the health of the lungs and even improve their performance. Always breathe in through the nose, as the nasal passages are equipped to warm, dampen and clean the air before it is taken into the lungs.

Incorrect breathing

Although breathing is a natural and automatic process, it is surprising how many people breathe incorrectly, using shallow movements in the top of the chest rather than using the full capacity of the lungs. Bad posture also affects breathing, as round shoulders and a cramped chest will lead to shallow breathing. Incorrect breathing can lead to and aggravate many problems, such as asthma, bronchitis, stomach and digestive problems. Remember too, that smoking affects the efficiency of the lungs and can lead to permanent lung damage. Many smokers find that when they take up regular exercise, their smoking decreases, enabling some to give up altogether.

Breathing and exercise

It is particularly important to breathe properly during exercise, especially when performing more 'aerobic' activities. 'Aerobic' simply means 'with air'; aerobic activities are endurance exercises which increase the body's capacity to carry oxygen to the working muscles and remove carbon dioxide and other toxic wastes.

Try to perform some form of more vigorous exercise every day to make yourself slightly breathless, and thereby increase the action

The action of the diaphragm

Breathing in

lungs fill with air

diaphragm moves down

abdomen is pushed out

Breathing out

air is expelled from lungs

diaphragm rises

abdomen flattens

of the heart and lungs. Why not run for the bus next time, or walk up the stairs instead of taking the lift?

Breathing and stress

One of the commonest causes of incorrect breathing is stress. Think of your first reaction to surprise, shock or fright – it is to take in a sharp gasp of air. This is a completely involuntary movement, but repeated over and over again, it leaves the diaphragm tight and the chest muscles constricted, often resulting in breathlessness. Next time you are feeling anxious, try taking a few good slow deep breaths. It will give you time to stop and assess your problem.

A word of warning here though. Do not take too many deep breaths, three or four will do – and then breathe normally, making sure that you are using your rib-cage. Too much deep breathing can upset the delicate breathing centre of the brain, and cause giddiness.

How to check your breathing

Exercise Stand or sit in front of a mirror, correct your posture and place your hands on your lower rib-cage, fingers touching in the centre. Breathe in deeply, keeping your hands against your ribs. Feel and watch the ribs expanding up and out to the sides as you fill your lungs with air, while your finger-tips separate as well. Your abdomen should also expand naturally. As you breathe out your ribs will fall, and your hands return to their previous position.

Watch your shoulders; they should only move very slightly. If they heave up and down and you feel little or no movement in the rib-cage, you are breathing shallowly in the top of the chest.

Practise this exercise three or four times a day until you feel you are breathing correctly.

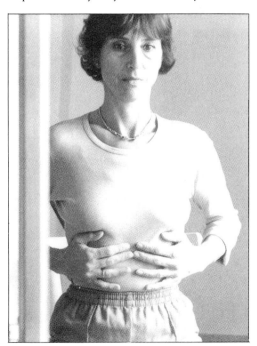 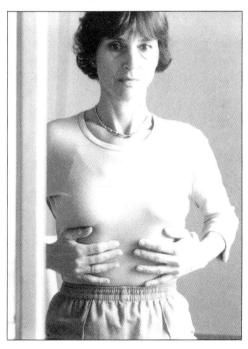

CHANGING POSITIONS

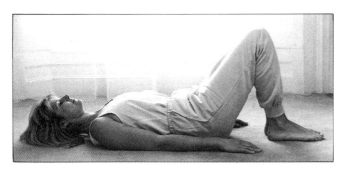

The abdominal muscles are less vulnerable than the back muscles and should always be used in conjunction with the arms to change your position from lying down to sitting up, or vice versa. This technique is essential if you have back problems.

As you get up off a chair or stool, practise developing your balance, using the strong muscles of your thighs to lift you up avoiding back strain.

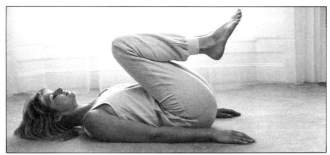

Lying to sitting

Bring your knees into your chest, roll over on to your right side (or left if you prefer), then, pushing up with your right elbow and left hand, sit up. (Reverse this for the left side.)

To lie down from sitting, turn sideways and lower yourself with your arms until you are lying on your side, then roll on to your back.

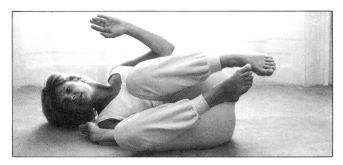

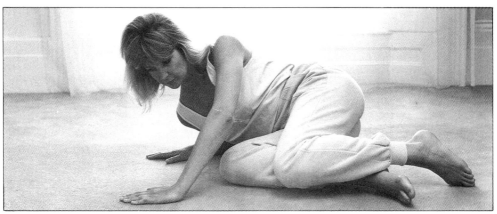

Sitting to standing

Place both feet quite close in to the chair, one foot slightly in front of the other, and leave your arms by your sides. Move to the edge of the chair and push up to standing with your thighs.

Do not use your hands to help you, but keep your back straight, head up and neck lengthened. Reverse the movement when sitting down again.

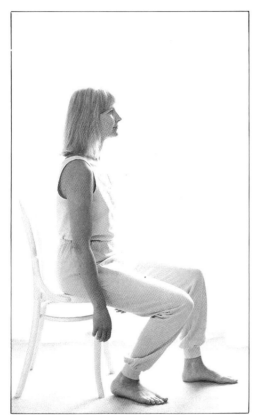
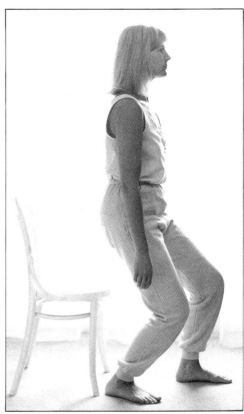

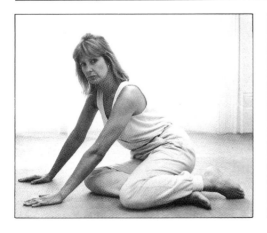
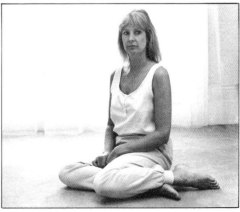

THE FACE

The muscles of the face and neck are quite complex and varied. Giving them a good squeeze and stretch will be beneficial, increasing the circulation to the muscles and skin, and improving both their tone and appearance.

Everyone uses their facial muscles in their own particular way, but this can lead to 'set' lines around the eyes, between the brows and around the mouth. Lines and wrinkles inevitably develop as we grow older, but there is quite a lot that can be done to improve muscle tone and therefore delay the worst of these for some time. Men tend to have better facial muscle tone than women; perhaps this is because they exercise their facial muscles each time they shave!

Neck firmer

Exercise Stick your lower jaw forward and move it strongly up and down, feeling the muscles of your neck tighten each time you bring your jaw up. Repeat as often as possible. This exercise is excellent for double chins – or preventing them!

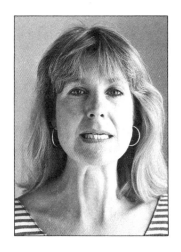

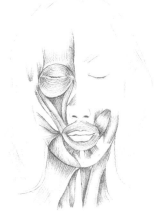

Outer layer   Inner layer
The face and neck muscles

Facial squeeze and stretch

Exercise Screw your face up tightly, pursing your mouth and closing your eyes tightly. Then open up your face, lifting your eyebrows, opening your eyes as wide as possible, stretching your mouth open and sticking out your tongue as far as it will go. Repeat eight times.

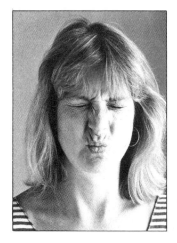

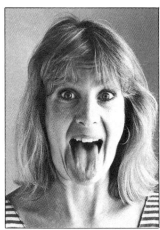

Chin wag

Exercise Drop your jaw, opening your mouth as you do so. Move your chin from left to right in a sliding action. Now repeat the action of the jaw with your mouth closed and your lips pursed, as if you were shaving. Repeat quite slowly eight times.

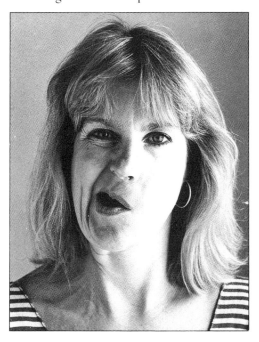 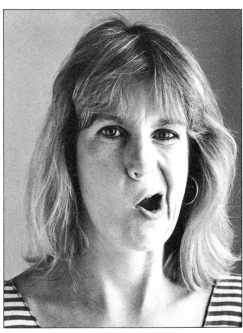

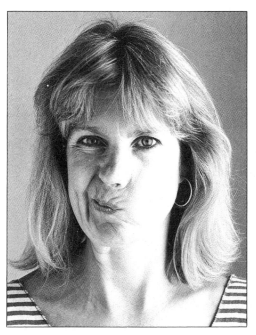 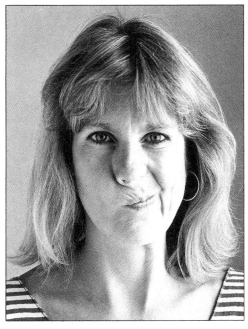

NECK AND SHOULDERS

The neck and shoulders are particularly vulnerable to stiffness and tension and it is important to release any tightness here before working on other parts of the body.

If you are not very fit and tire easily, the first set of exercises may be performed sitting down. As you become stronger do them standing up. This will help to increase your stamina and is good for the balance.

Try to prevent tension building up in the neck and shoulder muscles by doing the following exercises every day.

Head rolling and turning

Exercise Sitting or standing correctly, first check your posture, then let your head fall forward. Feel the weight of your head stretching out the muscles at the back of the neck. Hold this position for as long as you need to release the tension.

Gently roll your head round towards the right shoulder, holding the stretch on the way in any position which feels particularly tight, and using your fingers to massage into the spot as you stretch. This will increase the circulation to the muscles. Repeat to the left.

Take your head back to the centre, lift it up and turn to look over your right shoulder and then the left. Repeat the whole exercise several times until your neck feels loose and free.

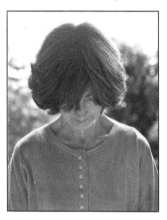 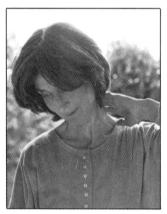 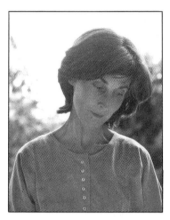

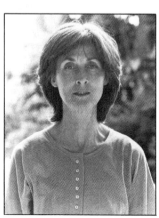 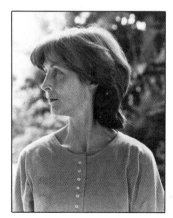 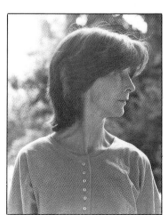

Shoulder lift

The shoulder girdle – collar bone and shoulder-blade – is a very mobile joint, which needs to be kept moving freely.
Exercise Lift your shoulders up towards your ears, then pull them back, squeezing the shoulder-blades together.

From this position drop your shoulders as far down as you can and release. Repeat eight times.

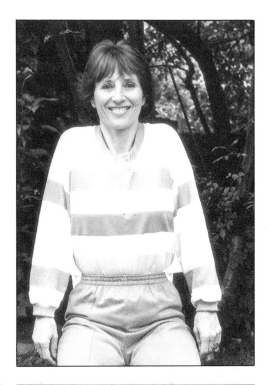

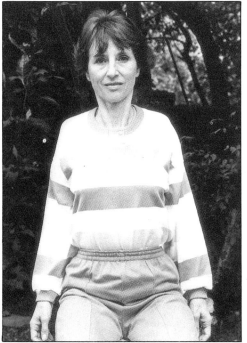

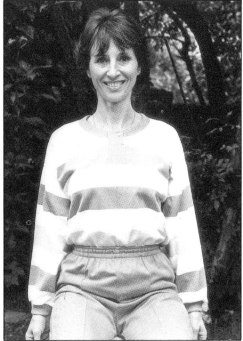

Shoulder circling

This exercise keeps the shoulder joints moving freely and the muscles of the shoulder area flexible. It increases the action of the heart and lungs, and is a very good way to warm up.

Exercise Place your hands on your shoulders and circle your elbows forward, up and back, making as wide a circle as possible.

Progression Fully extend your right arm and circle it from the shoulder, up and back, brushing your ear with your upper arm and reaching as far as possible behind you. Repeat with the left arm, then circle both arms together, taking care not to arch your back. Repeat each of these exercises eight times.

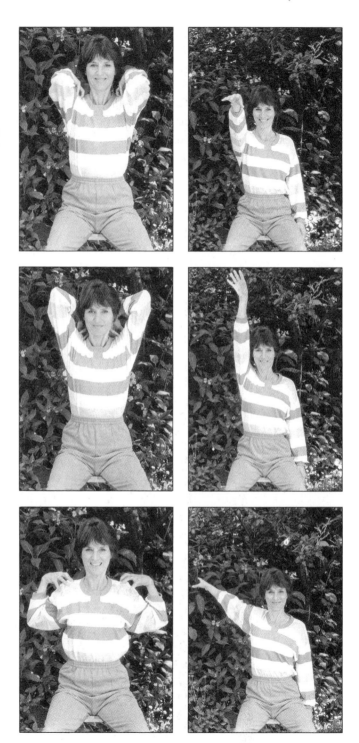

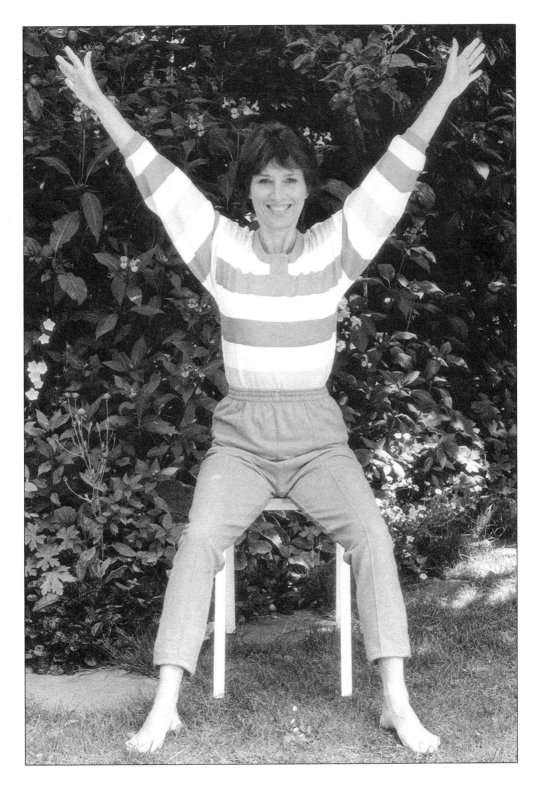

Self-massage

Self-massage can be used when you have completed the other neck and shoulder exercises, or is useful if you have not had time to do the exercises and feel tense in this area.

The shoulders Take your right hand over your left shoulder, feel gently with your finger tips for any tender spot and massage into it. Then take hold of the shoulder muscle firmly with your fist, rather as you would pick up a cat by the scruff of its neck, and circle the shoulder slowly up, back and down, several times. Repeat on the other side.

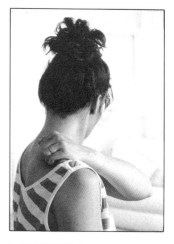

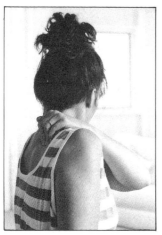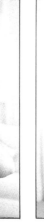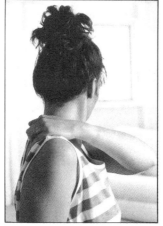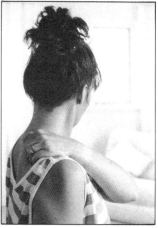

The neck Take hold of the skin at the back of the neck in the same way and gently nod your head up and down.

Finish off by firmly circling your finger-tips down your neck and shoulders.

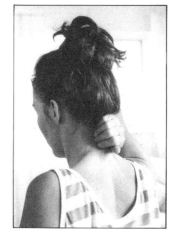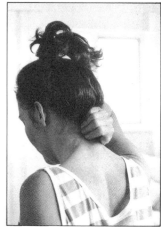

ARMS AND HANDS

Apart from the face, no other area of the body gives away age more than the arms. Wearing sleeveless dresses can become an embarrassment if the skin texture becomes pimply, and the muscles slacken, especially those under the upper arm.

Strength in the arm muscles is important in order to continue carrying out everyday activities without tiring unnecessarily. Even simple movements such as carrying the shopping basket, a watering can or a small child are made easier. Working on strengthening and firming the arm muscles will also increase the circulation and greatly improve the appearance and texture of the skin.

The hands too can benefit from exercise. As we grow older, the finger joints can become stiff, making it increasingly difficult to stretch them and use them properly. For this reason, arthritis often starts in the finger joints. Keeping the fingers flexible will help with the many movements performed with the fingers: lifting, carrying, writing, typing, sewing, gardening, even tying shoe-laces, brushing your hair or holding a cup of coffee.

Full arm stretch

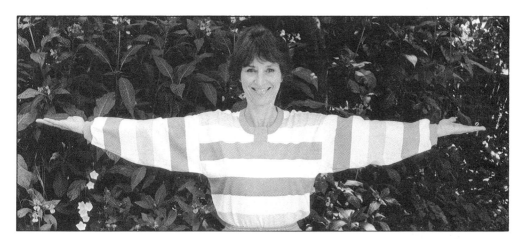

Any exercise you perform with your arms outstretched will strengthen them and increase your stamina.

Exercise Start by warming up the elbow joints. Stretch your arms out to the sides at shoulder level, palms up. Bend your elbows and bring your hands to your shoulders, then stretch out your arms again. If you feel any tension in your neck allow your head to fall forward. Repeat eight times and release.

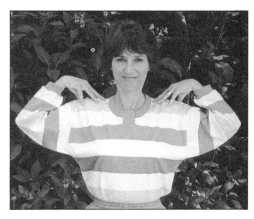

Under-arm stretch and wrist mobilizer

Exercise Stretch your arms straight out in front of you, at shoulder level. Flex your hands strongly, feeling the stretch under your arms, and then drop your hands from the wrists. Repeat eight times.

Without dropping your arms, circle your hands from the wrists, eight times in each direction.

Release and give your hands a good shake.

Finger flexing and stretching

This keeps the finger joints flexible.
Exercise Make loose fists with your hands and then open them, stretching the fingers as wide apart as possible. Hold for a moment and then repeat eight times.

On the last stretch, circle your thumb, first one way then the other. It should move freely with no pain or clicking in the joint. Repeat eight times.

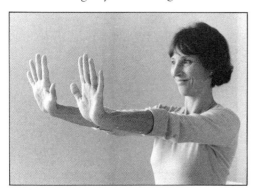 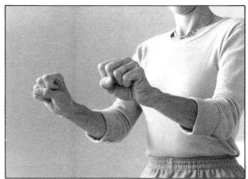

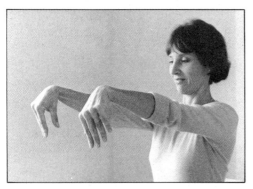 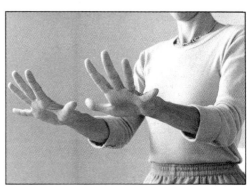

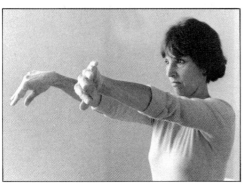 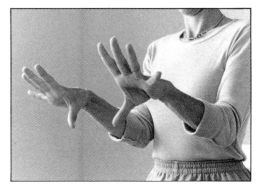

Arm and shoulder strengthener

This exercise strengthens your arms and works into the muscles between the shoulder blades.
Exercise Take your arms out to your sides, making loose fists with your hands; check that you have dropped your shoulders away from your ears. Remember to maintain correct posture; keep your back straight and do not allow your lower back to arch.

Pull your arms back to squeeze the shoulder blades together. Holding this contraction push back firmly with your arms. If you feel the contraction is a strain on the neck, let your head come forward. Push back and release eight times.

Progression As you grow stronger you can repeat the exercise for longer and add variations by making small circles with your arms, or lifting them up and down within a small range. Keep squeezing the shoulder blades together throughout the exercise, and breathe well.

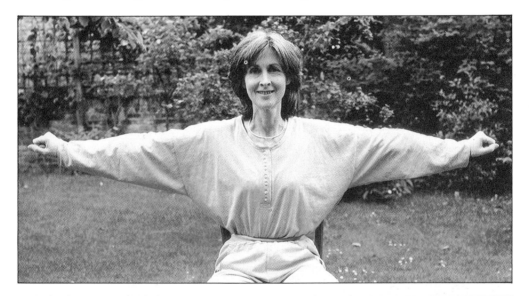

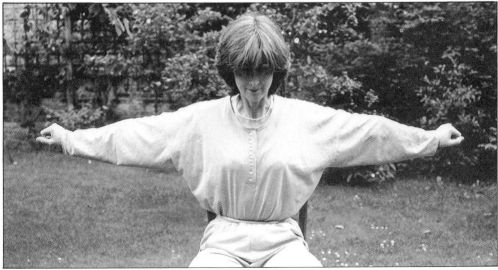

Shoulder squeeze

This exercise will open and lift the chest and squeeze the muscles between the shoulder blades. It is an excellent treatment for round shoulders, especially if you are also practising correct posture, and also strengthens the muscles at the top of the arms.

Exercise Clasp your hands behind you, interlocking your fingers, and rest them on your lower back, elbows bent. Squeeze the elbows towards each other, and release; repeat eight times.

Try to synchronize your breathing during the exercise, breathing out as you squeeze your elbows together, and breathing in as you release.

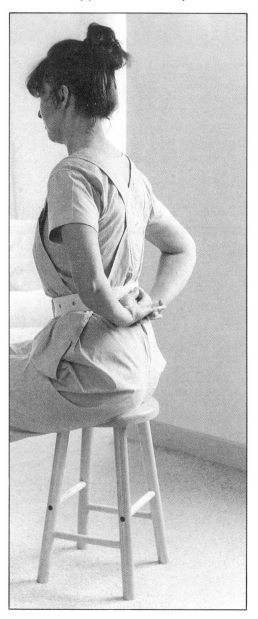
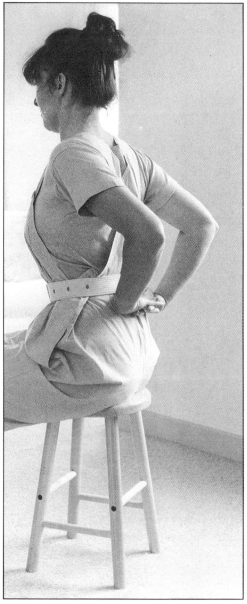

Progression From the previous position, straighten your arms out behind you keeping your hands clasped together, then lift and lower them. Do not allow the body to tip forward. This exercise will stretch the muscles in your arms and help to get rid of any stiffness in the shoulder joints.

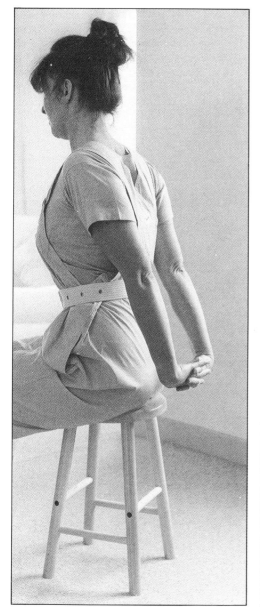
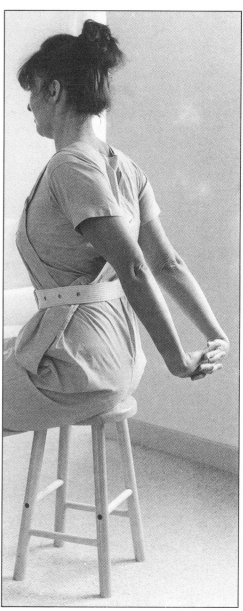

Final stretch

Finish this set of arm and hand exercises with a good stretch.

Sitting exercise Sit on a firm chair or stool and roll your pelvis so that the pubic bone lifts upwards. Stretch out your arms, hands clasped and palms away from you, straighten the knees and flex the feet. Breathe well. You should feel a good stretch across the back of the shoulders and down the spine and backs of the legs. Then release, sitting normally again.

Breathe in and as you breathe out, repeat the stretch.

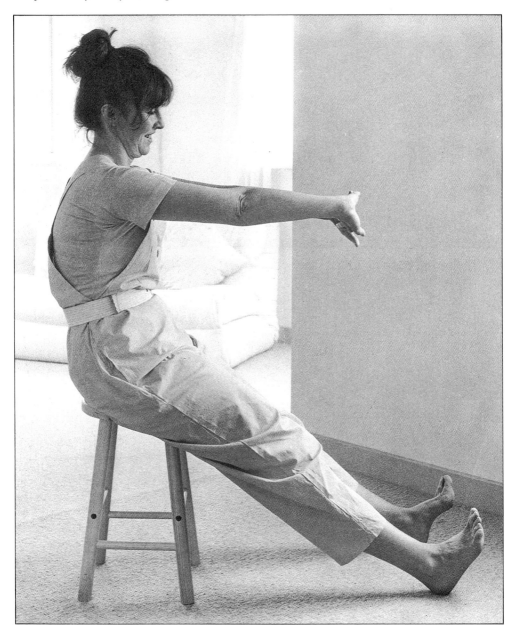

Standing exercise Stand up straight, bend your knees and tip your pelvis back, pulling in the abdominal muscles and stretching your arms away from you. Straighten up again, breathe in gently and repeat on the out breath.

You can do these exercises with a partner. Ask her to pull firmly on your arms as you stretch.

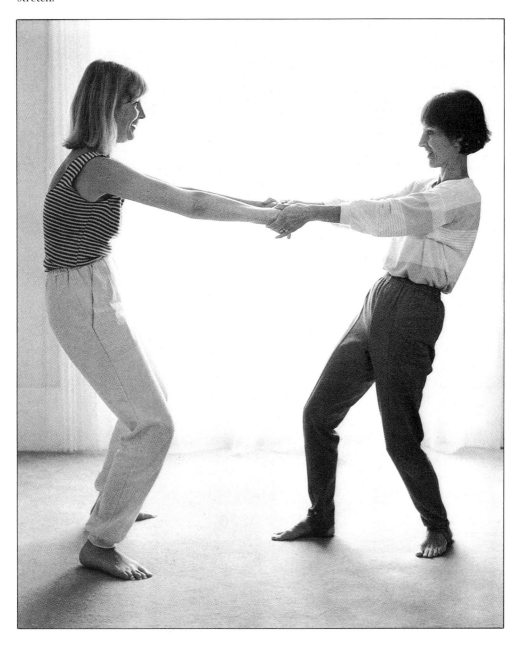

THE ABDOMINAL MUSCLES

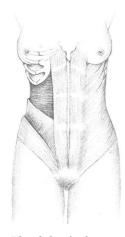

The muscles of the abdomen are rather like a corset, running vertically from the breast-bone and ribs down to the pubic bone, diagonally from the ribs to the mid-line (a strip of fibrous tissue called the linea alba), and horizontally from the spine round to the mid-line.

All sets of muscles work in pairs, one contracting, the other stretching to allow for movement, but if one set becomes weak, its opposite has to work more strongly to compensate. In this way, weak abdominal muscles put a lot of strain on the lower back, which can lead to back pain and other problems.

Strong abdominal muscles are essential for good posture (see p. 68) and the support of the spine. Conversely, bad posture can lead to weak abdominal muscles. If you stand with a sway-back your lower back is over-arched, pushing the stomach forward. Similarly, if you slouch, the abdominal muscles become slack and stick out.

A 'spare tyre' can be improved by good posture. Stretch your

The abdominal muscles

Positions for abdominal exercises

Some abdominal exercises can be done lying on the floor. Others can be done sitting or standing. You might like to start doing them sitting, then progress to standing when you are stronger, remembering to maintain correct posture throughout.

Before you start any of the waist exercises, sitting or standing, move your legs further apart. Rest your hands on your shoulders or clasp them to the back of the head. Then begin the exercise.

As you become stronger, you can circle your arms above your head. Make sure that you do not arch your back. Pull your shoulders down away from your ears.

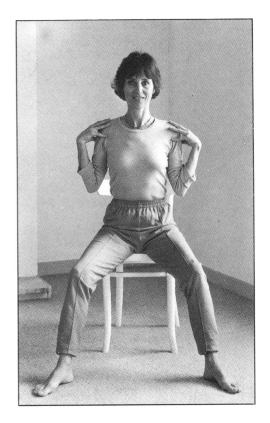

arms above your head – notice how your waist tightens and your tummy flattens.

There are a wide variety of exercises which strengthen the abdominal muscles but there are two golden rules to follow to ensure that you are doing them properly.

The first is to breathe correctly. In order to strengthen the muscles, you must contract them. When you breathe in your abdominal muscles will stretch and expand under the pressure of the air in your lungs and it is self-defeating to try to contract against this pressure. It can also increase blood pressure and put pressure on the pelvic floor. So remember always to breathe *out* as you contract your abdominal muscles to perform the exercise.

The second rule is to make sure that you start with a good pelvic tilt and maintain it while doing the curl-up or curl-down exercises. This will protect your lower back. Tilt your pelvis so that your pubic bone moves up towards your face as you breathe out. You can practise this movement sitting on a stool or lying on the floor. The simple action of rolling the pelvis and contracting the abdominal muscles is enough to strengthen them.

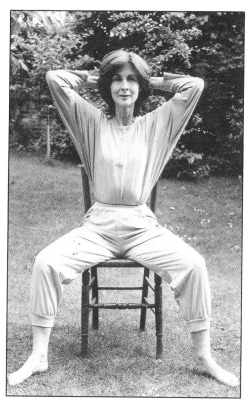
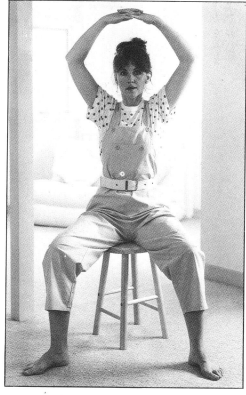

Side bends

This exercise stretches and strengthens the muscles at the side of the waist and mobilizes the spine.

Exercise Bring your arms up to one of the positions already described, breathe in gently and as you breathe out bend over to the right, lifting the rib-cage and lengthening over to that side.

Move in eight small further stretches, hold the position as far over to the side as possible for a moment, breathe in and return to the centre. Repeat on the other side.

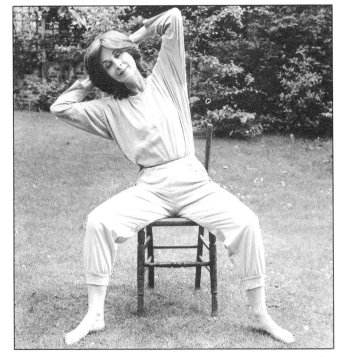

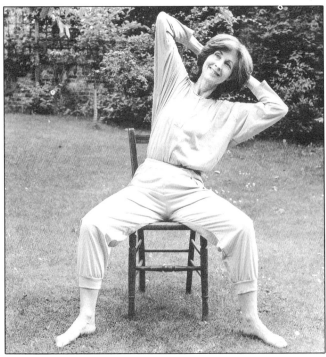

Waist twists

To work the diagonal muscles of the waist you need to use a twist, but this must be done with great care. If you have any history of back trouble do not try this exercise. If you feel any pain or discomfort as you do the exercise, stop at once.

Exercise Sit on a firm chair or stool. (A stool is best since there is no back to impede your movement.) Place your feet flat on the floor and fairly wide apart. Correct your posture.

Place your hands on your shoulders, elbows relaxed by your sides, shoulders down. Gently twist round to the right, looking over your shoulder, then work in small further movements until you are as far round as possible. Hold the twist, breathing well. Make sure that the top half of your body is immediately above your hips – not leaning forward or out. You should aim to have your shoulders at 90° to your hips as you hold the twist, but work carefully towards this position.

Return slowly to the centre and repeat on the other side.

Compare each side of the body as you work – you will probably find that you can twist round further on one side than the other. Work harder on your tighter side to balance the body so that it is working evenly.

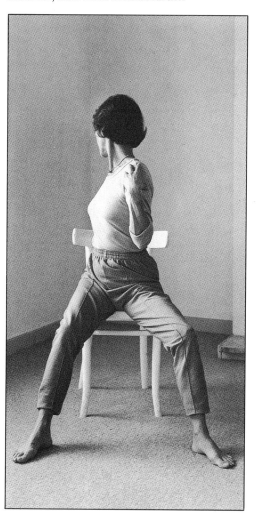
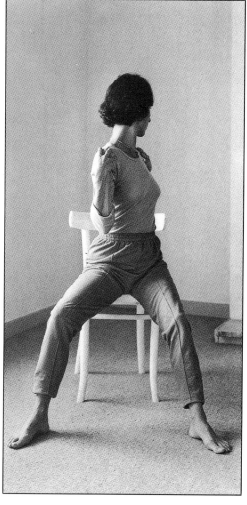

Progression Standing, cross your arms and hold them away from you at shoulder level. Bend your knees and gently twist round to the right, keeping both hips facing forwards. Hold the twist for a moment, return to the centre and repeat on the other side.

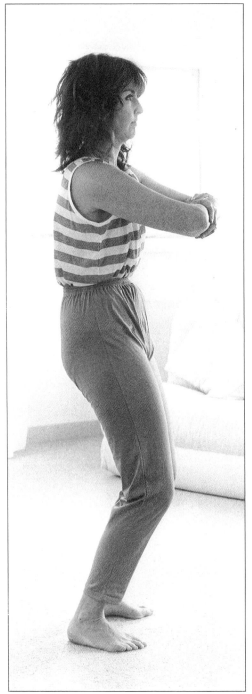

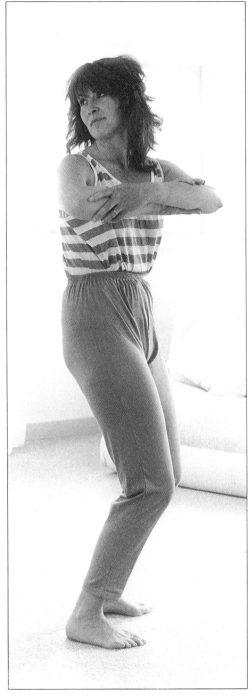

Releasing swing

This exercise can be done immediately after the standing waist twists. It is very good for the balance.

Exercise Release your arms and let them fall away from the body. Keeping your knees bent, swing your body slowly from side to side, allowing the arms to follow the movement.

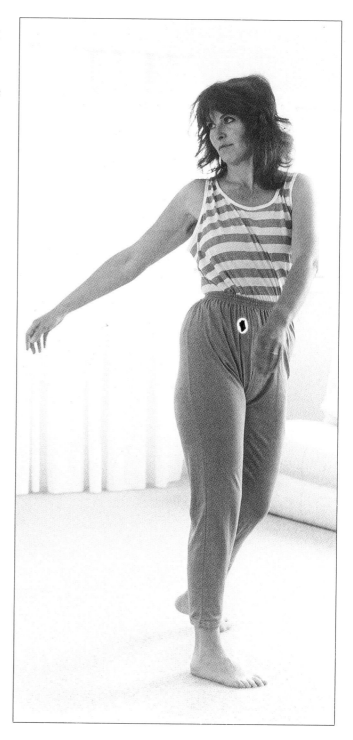

Diagonal twist

This exercise works the diagonal muscles of the waist and the lower back. If you feel any pain or discomfort in your lower back as you do this exercise, stop at once.

Exercise Lie flat on the floor, shoulders down away from the ears. Bring your knees into your chest and stretch your arms out to the sides at shoulder level.

Keeping your thighs as close to your ribs as possible, roll your legs over to the right, turning your head to the left as you do so. Lift the legs to the centre and roll them to the other side, head turning to the right. Continue to roll from side to side for as long as is comfortable, and try to work up a nice rhythm to the exercise. Do not let your legs drop away from your body as this will strain your lower back. Make sure that your shoulders stay flat on the floor to ensure that you get a good twist from the waist.

To finish off, roll to one side and hold the twist for a few moments, breathing well. Repeat on the other side.

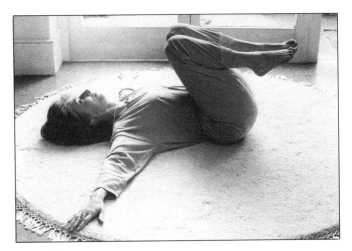

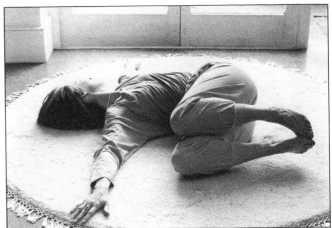

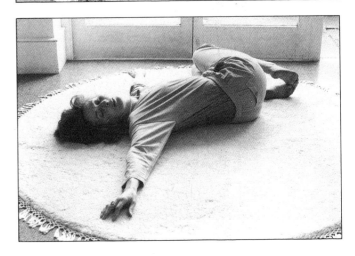

Curl-down

The following exercises work the vertical abdominal muscles.

Exercise Sit with a straight back, your legs hip-width apart and the knees bent, feet flat on the floor. Place your hands under your thighs.

Breathe in, and as you breathe out roll the top of the pelvis back, bringing your pubic bone up, tightening your abdominal muscles as you do so. Keep your shoulders down and your head tilted forward. Hold for a moment, then sit up slowly. Repeat eight times.

Progression Tilt your pelvis, tighten your abdominal muscles and, rounding your back, slowly curl down. (Your tummy should not bulge or quiver – if it does you are straining. Go back to the easier part of the exercise and strengthen your muscles further that way before progressing again.)

Hold for as long as is comfortable, taking small shallow breaths, and then slowly uncurl and sit upright. If you feel any strain in your back you are not working your abdominal muscles correctly and are trying to roll down too far, so go back to the easier exercise.

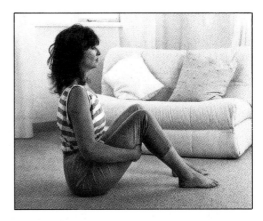

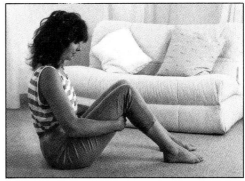

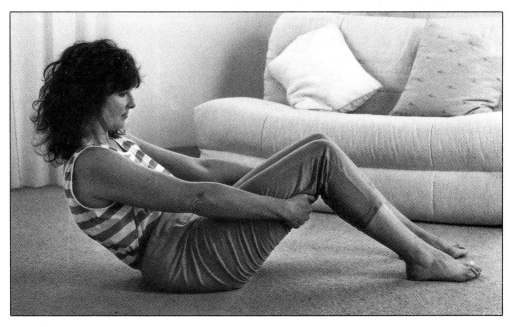

Advanced curl-down

This is a stronger version of the previous exercise.
Exercise Fold your arms in front of you as you roll back, keeping your shoulders down. If you feel any strain in the neck turn your head from side to side, keeping it tilted forwards.

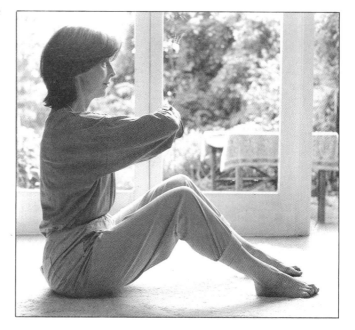

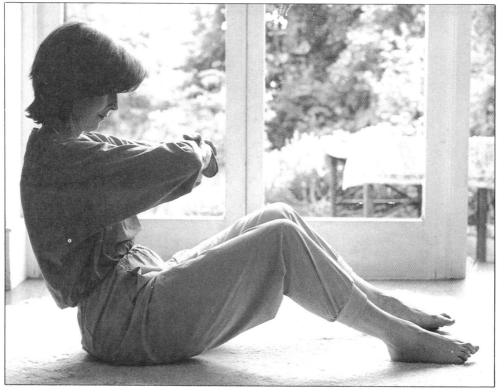

Progression As you grow stronger still, clasp your hands behind your head as you roll down, but do not attempt this until you are confident that the abdominal muscles are really strong.

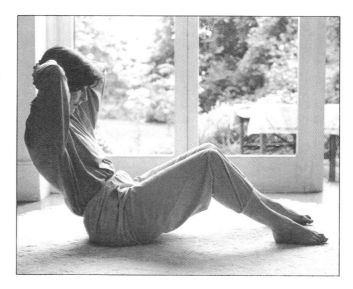

Spine stretch

Finish off the curl-down exercises by stretching your spine.
Exercise Sit on the floor with the soles of your feet together. Push them away from you, keeping your knees slightly bent.

Round your back, allowing your head to hang forwards to stretch your neck. Stretch forwards, clasping your hands round your feet and breathing well. Hold for a few moments and uncurl slowly.

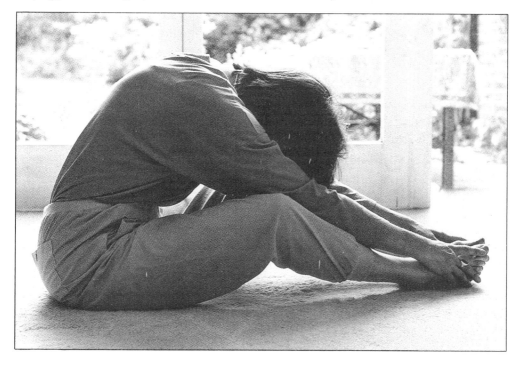

Curling up

Use of a stool to support the legs helps to keep the pelvis tilted during this exercise.
Exercise Lie on your back with a cushion under your head and rest your legs over a chair or stool. Breathe in and as you breathe out, tilt the pelvis up, tighten the abdominal muscles and lift your head and shoulders from the floor, stretching forward with your arms. Keep your chin tucked in and shoulders down. (If this is very hard for you hold on to the backs of your thighs to help you lift up.) Repeat this six times.
Progression Lift yourself up higher with arms stretched forward, then lift and lower yourself within a short range four times, then lower slowly back down to the floor. Remember to maintain the pelvic tilt and tight abdominal muscles throughout the exercise.

If you feel any strain in the neck, roll your head from side to side when you release to the floor. Repeat six times.

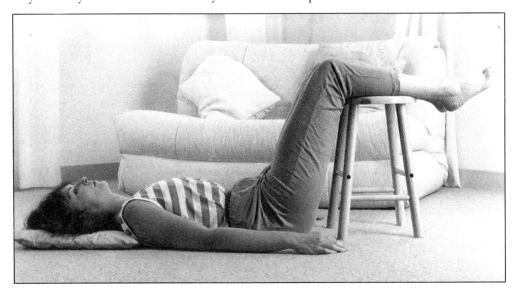

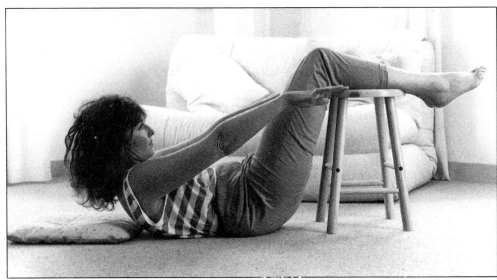

THE BACK

The muscles and vertebrae

The muscles of the back support the spine, and, together with the abdominals, the whole upper torso. In order to maintain good posture it is important that back muscles should be strong and flexible. They are arranged in layers, similar to the corset of the abdominals, to enable the back to move in several ways – bending to the side, forwards, twisting and bending backwards.

The spine is composed of bones, or vertebrae, and discs between the vertebrae which act as shock-absorbers and allow for movement, forming a cushion between the vertebrae. Weak back muscles, together with the possible deterioration of the discs and vertebrae as we grow older, can lead to the discs being compressed or even 'slipping' out, causing backache and sometimes severe pain. Gradual strengthening of the back muscles can help to avoid back problems and even to alleviate existing ones.

Working on the back

A good way to work on the back muscles is to sit on the floor. If you find it difficult to sit freely with a straight back use all the props and aids you need to help you and dispense with them as you grow stronger. You could work with a partner who could correct your posture by placing a hand against your back. If you are working on your own use a mirror to start with to check that your back is always straight.

You may find when you try the following exercises for the first time that one is easier than the others. This will depend on the flexibility of the hip joints and the stretch in your thigh muscles. If you feel any pain do not continue. Learn to distinguish between stretch and pain so that you can progress with the exercises, avoiding unnecessary discomfort or injury.

The back muscles

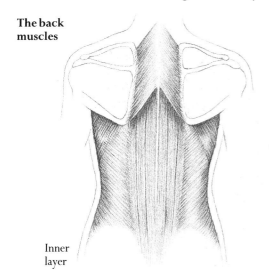

Inner layer

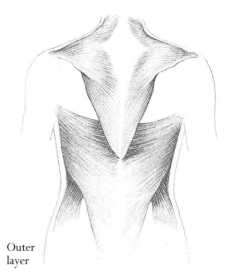

Outer layer

Back strengthener

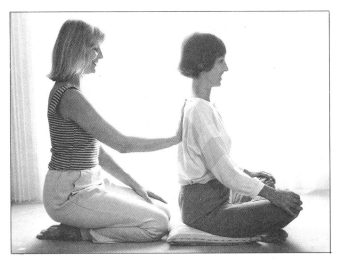 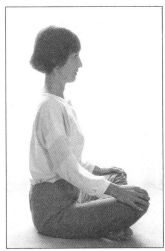

Exercise Sit cross-legged up against a wall or sofa and make sure that your back is flat against it. The back of your head should rest against the support, with the neck long and your chin tucked slightly in. Pull your shoulders down and rest your hands comfortably on your knees. If you find it difficult to keep your pelvis centred, sit on a small cushion to correct it. Breathe well and try to lift and lengthen your body upwards to stretch your spine.

Practise sitting in this position as often as you can. When your back has strengthened and it becomes easier, dispense with the cushion and sit with a straight back, unsupported, for as long as is comfortable.

Progression Using the cushion and support if you need them, sit with the soles of your feet together, which has the added bonus of loosening your hip joints and inside thigh muscles.

Further progression Dispense with the cushion and support and, holding on to your feet or ankles, bend forward slowly from the hips to an angle of about 45°, keeping your back straight. Keep your chin tucked in and lead with your forehead to keep your neck lengthened. Hold the stretch for a few moments, release and then stretch forward again.

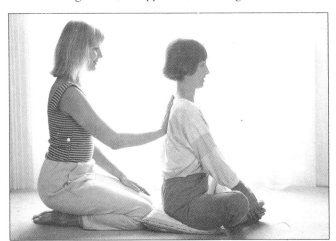 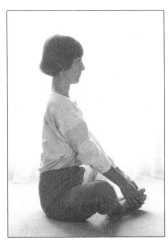

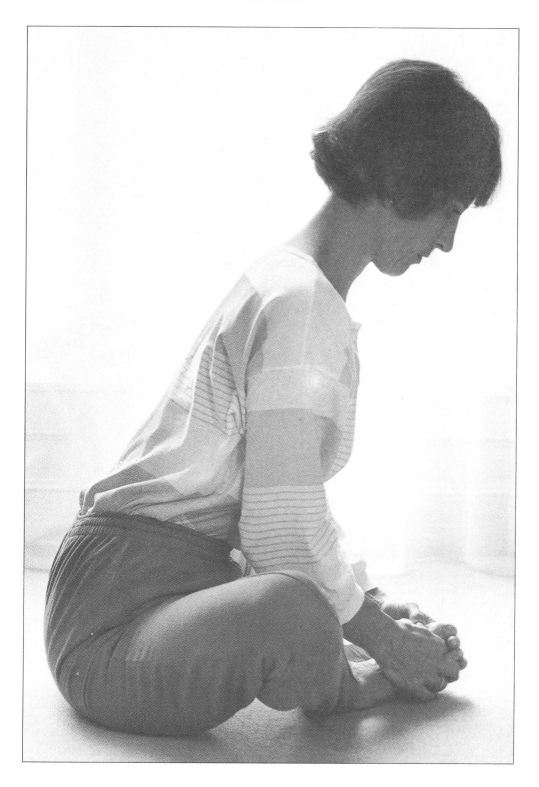

Back strengthener and hamstring stretch

Exercise Sit against a support on a cushion and push your legs out in front of you, feet together and knees straight. Flex your feet strongly and tighten the muscles on the front of the thighs. You should feel a good stretch along the backs of the legs. To help straighten your back, place a belt or scarf round your feet, pull gently on it to help you lift and lengthen your spine.

Progression Move away from the support when you feel strong enough, but continue to use the belt around your feet. Breathe well and keep your spine lengthened. When you can sit in this position without the cushion and with your pelvis centred, bend forwards from the hips, keeping a straight back, the neck long.

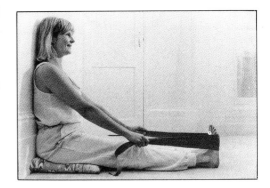

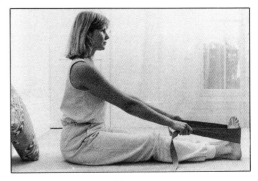

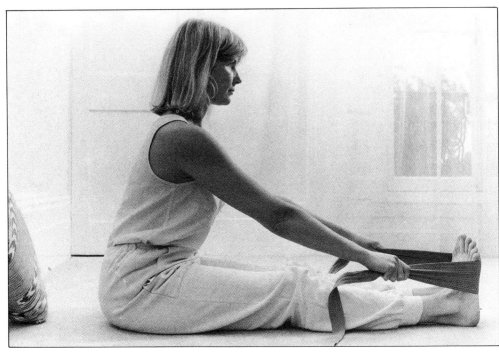

Back strengthener and inside-thigh stretch

This exercise stretches the inside thigh muscles
and loosens the hip joints as well as
strengthening the back.
Exercise Using the support and cushion, sit
straight with legs wide apart and again place a
belt or scarf around each foot to help you. Flex
them and feel the stretch on your inside thighs.
Progression Move away from the support,
dispense with the cushion and finally bend
forward from the hips, keeping the back
straight.

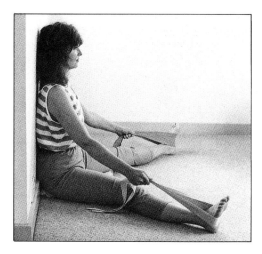

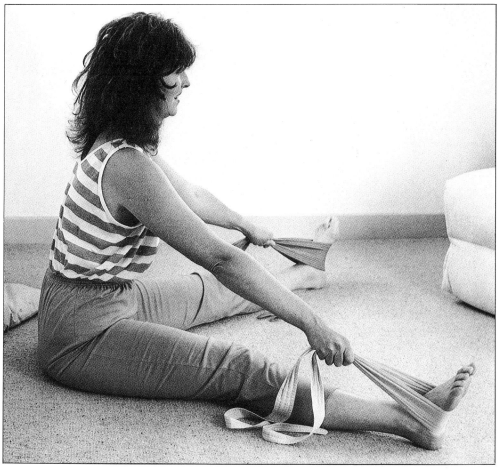

BUTTOCKS AND THIGHS

Of all the areas of the body to come under scrutiny, probably the one that many people are most concerned about are the buttocks and thighs. A sedentary life-style and an increase in weight are two common factors which contribute to a spreading in this area, particularly as we grow older; the buttock muscles drop, and together with flabby thigh muscles, spread to the sides to form the so-called 'pear-shaped bottom'. Thighs and buttocks are also prone to pimples or prominent hair follicles, which are due to poor circulation.

Exercise will tighten and firm the muscles, lifting the buttocks and toning up the thighs, and the increase in circulation brought about by exercise will greatly improve the appearance of the skin.

A very simple but effective buttock and thigh exercise (which is also impossible to illustrate!) is to squeeze the buttocks firmly together, holding the contraction for a count of two and then releasing; repeat as often as you like.

Outside thigh strengthener

This exercise strengthens and firms the muscles on the outside of the thighs.
Exercise Lie on your side, stretched out into a straight line, and rest your head on your hand. Place the other hand next to your chest for balance. Bend the leg nearest the floor slightly. With the toes and knee of the top leg turned forwards and the foot flexed, raise it into the air a little way. Keep your hips one above the other and make sure you are still in a straight line.

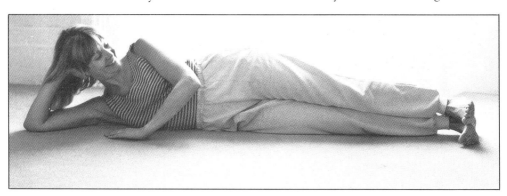

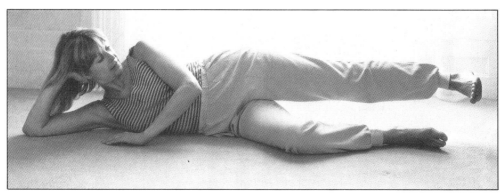

Working the muscles Lift the upper leg higher into the air and slowly lower it halfway; do not let it drop back on to the other leg. Continue lifting and lowering slowly and deliberately eight times to begin with, building up to more as you grow stronger. Do not just wave your leg up and down – feel the muscles on the outside of your thigh working as they lift the weight of your leg. Keep breathing well throughout.

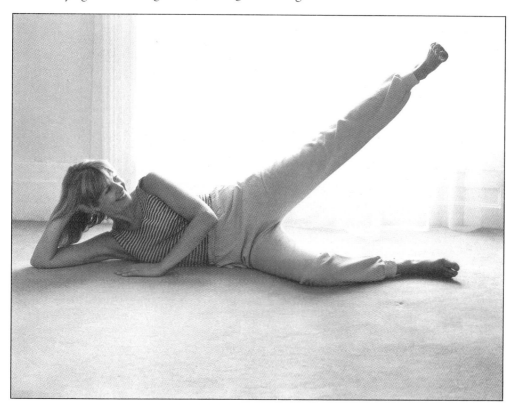

To finish When you have done as many repeats as you can without strain, lower your leg to the floor. Keeping your head and arm in the same position, bend the knee into your chest. Take a deep breath and give your thigh a good rub.

Roll over on to your other side and repeat with the other leg. Remember to keep breathing deeply.

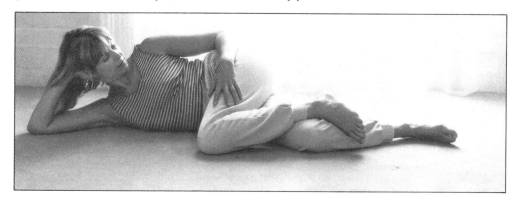

Buttock squeeze with pelvic tilt

This exercise firms and strengthens the buttocks and thighs.

Exercise Lie on the floor with your legs hip-width apart, knees bent, feet flat on the floor. If you find that your chin pokes up towards the ceiling place a cushion under your head.

Breathe in and as you breathe out, push your lower back into the floor, rolling the pelvis up so that the pubic bone comes towards your face. Tighten the buttock muscles together. Release and repeat eight times. Roll the pelvis down, take a deep breath, then release.

Progression Roll the pelvis further up so that the buttocks come off the floor, but take care not to arch your lower back. Holding the pelvic tilt and pulling in your abdominal muscles, bring your knees together as you squeeze the buttocks, taking them apart as you release. This will tighten the muscles of the inside thighs too. Repeat eight times, then roll your back slowly down again, one vertebrae at a time to control the movement.

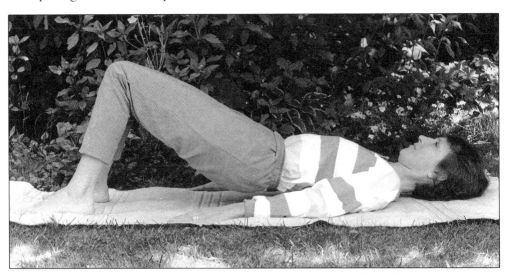

Knee-to-chest stretch

This exercise stretches the lower back and buttock muscles, and should be used immediately after the previous exercises.

Exercise Bring your knees into your chest, taking hold of each one separately. Breathe in and as you breathe out, gently draw your knees down towards the shoulders on either side, pressing your lower back into the floor to keep your back straight. Repeat several times, breathing well.

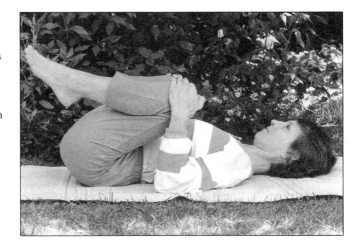

LEGS AND FEET

The muscles on the front of the thighs – the quadriceps – work the hip and knee joints, assisting each step that you take. If you allow the muscles to weaken these joints will suffer and your thighs may become fat and flabby with poor circulation, giving a pitted 'orange peel' appearance.

Another common problem with the legs is tight hamstrings. These muscles run down the back of the thighs and when tight can be associated with weak lower back muscles.

The muscles of the calves are responsible for the spring in your step which keeps you agile. These too can shorten and suffer from tightness, particularly if you wear high-heeled shoes. When the Achilles tendon at the base of the calf becomes too tight, sudden movement may cause injury. It is important to work on both the front and

back of the legs, for strong flexible leg muscles are important for maintaining good posture and ease of movement.

Older women often suffer from varicose veins, cramp and puffiness around the ankles but these conditions can be helped through exercise, which increases the circulation to the legs and feet, keeping them flexible and the joints mobile. Flexibility of the feet and ankles also gives lightness to walking.

The exercises given here for the legs and feet are best done sitting down. If you do them standing up, several have to be performed on one leg and then the other, and this can put considerable strain on the knee joints. When the muscles are stronger you can attempt the exercises standing up, but take care not to tire the supporting leg.

Knee bends

If you feel any pain in your back or knees, stop at once. Begin by sitting on a stool or chair.
Exercise Roll your pelvis back and pull in your abdominal muscles. Lift one leg, turn it out, flex

the foot and gently bend and straighten the leg, fully extending the knee and tightening the thigh muscles each time. Repeat eight times with each leg.

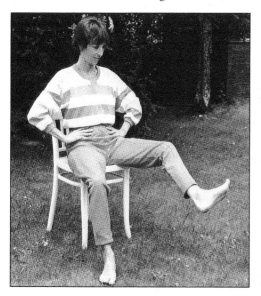
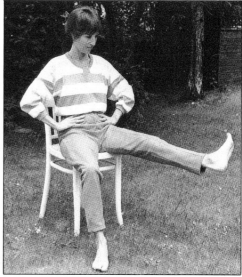

Ankle circling

When you first start working on your feet you may find that they feel stiff and it is difficult to co-ordinate the movements. Persevere with the exercises and you will soon notice the improved flexibility in your feet, ankles and toes. This ankle circling mobilizes the ankle joints.

Exercise Lift one leg towards your chest and hold on to your thigh. Try to keep your back as straight as possible. Circle the foot from the ankle, making as wide a movement as possible, eight times in each direction. Repeat with the other leg.

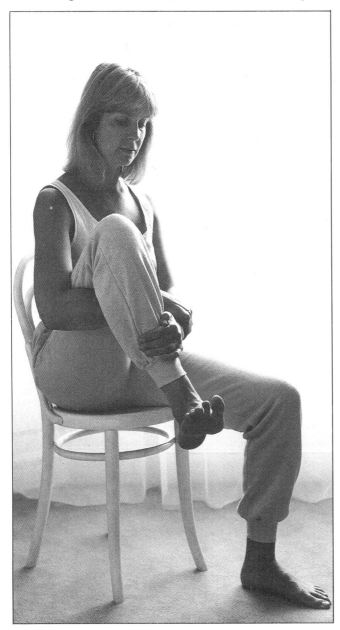

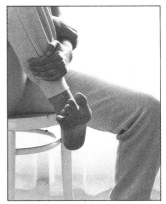

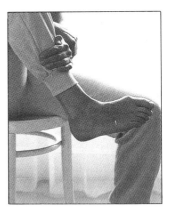

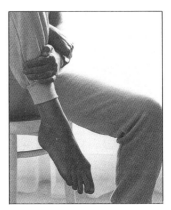

Foot mobilizer

This exercise helps to keep the feet flexible and also tones the muscles of the calf and shin. **Exercise** Put both feet forwards, hip-width apart and flex them strongly from the ankle joint, bringing your toes towards you. Now point the toes to stretch the ankles. Repeat eight times.

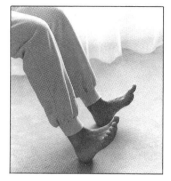 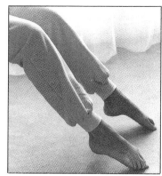

Arch strengtheners

The foot has two arches: the instep, and the metatarsal arch, which runs just below the toes. It is the flexibility of these arches which maintains the spring in your step. **Exercises** To strengthen the metatarsal arch, practise picking up a pencil with your toes.

To strengthen the instep, place both feet on the floor and, keeping the toes flat, draw them in towards the heel to lift the instep. Release and repeat four times.

If you find this exercise difficult, work each foot separately to begin with.

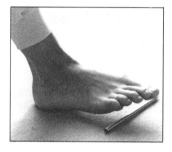 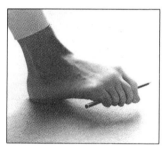

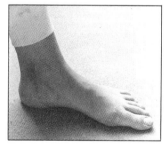 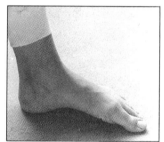

Toe stretch

Whenever you are barefoot, practise spreading your toes apart as wide as possible.

Finish off this series of exercises by shaking each foot loosely from the ankle. When you get up from your chair, remember to use your thighs rather than your back and arms (see p. 75).

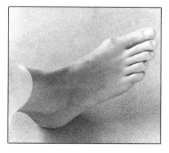 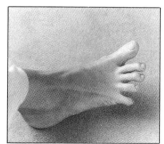

Calf strengthener

This exercise must be done standing up, but you can use a suitable support to keep your balance. Try to find a support that is high enough for you to maintain correct posture throughout the exercise. It strengthens the calf muscles and increases the circulation in the legs.
Exercise Hold on to a bar or work top for balance. Put your feet together and rise up on to the balls of the feet, keeping your heels pressed

together. Notice how your toes spread apart when you do this.

Lower your heels to the floor and lift up again, keeping your knees straight. Start gently and then bounce up each time. Repeat until you feel the muscles start to ache.

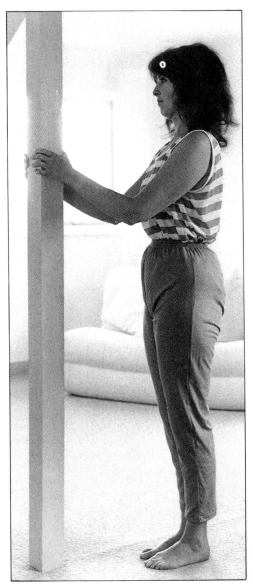
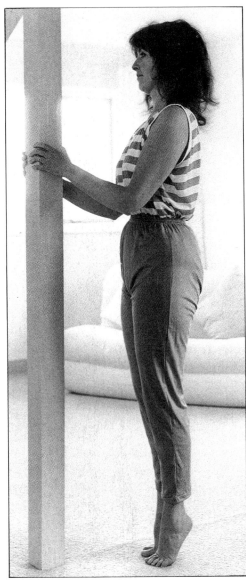

Progression To increase your heart and lung activity, hold on to the support and, without actually lifting your feet off the ground, run on the spot. Start by moving gently from one foot to the other and then speed it up. Make sure that you use the whole foot as you run, rippling through from the toes, the balls of the feet and down on to the heel each time. As one knee bends, straighten the other.

Continue for as long as you can until your legs begin to ache or you start to feel breathless.

Calf stretch

This exercise is designed to stretch the calf muscles, and can be used after either of the previous exercises. If you have been wearing high-heeled shoes over a number of years, your calf muscles may be very tight, so work carefully.

Exercise Hold on to the support. Keep your legs hip-width apart, pelvis forward. Take your right leg back, pressing the heel into the floor. You should feel a good stretch but no pain.

Tuck in your buttocks and gently push your body forward to increase the stretch. Start with small further movements and then hold the stretch for as long as possible. Repeat with the other leg, then both together.

Practise this stretch as often as possible around the house or office. Work tops, desks and basins are usually the ideal height.

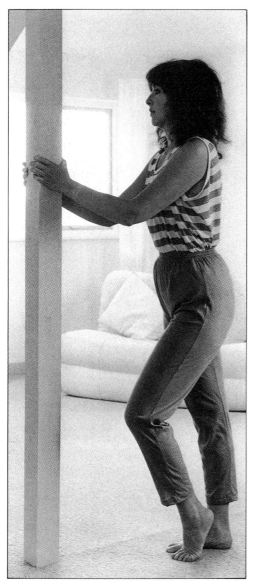

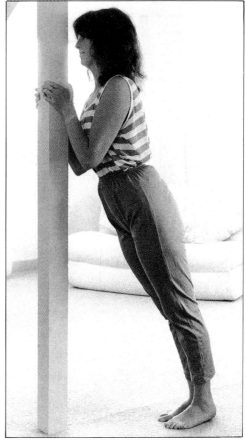

Improving your balance

This exercise requires a support that is the right height to maintain correct posture.

Exercise Stand with your hands on a support, feet hip-width apart. Lift up on to the balls of the feet, take your hands away and balance.

Progression Repeat the above movement, but lift your hands above your head and then balance.

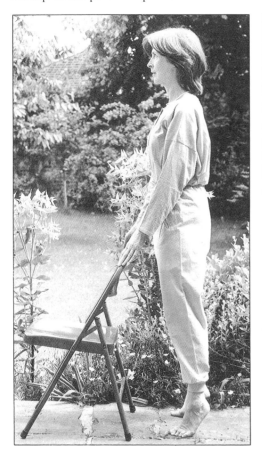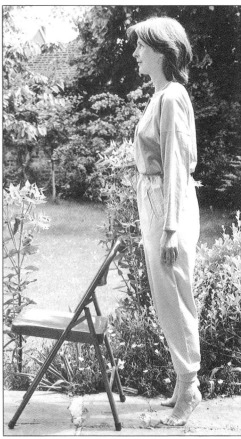

Foot massage

This is a marvellous all-round foot exercise which is particularly good for the relief of cramp in the feet and toes. You will need a small ball such as a squash ball for best results.

The exercise is best done standing up, but can be done sitting, if you prefer.

Exercise Stand up straight and correct your posture, keeping your arms relaxed by your sides.

Place a small firm ball under one foot and roll it around to massage the whole of the sole of the foot. Make sure you go into all the nooks and crannies – under the toes, down the sides of the foot, through the instep to the heel. Continue rolling for at least two minutes or longer.

When you have worked on one foot, stop and compare each side of the body. You should feel much more alive and stretched on the side you have been working. You may notice that your shoulder has dropped and the arm feels longer on that side.

Work on the other foot to balance the body.

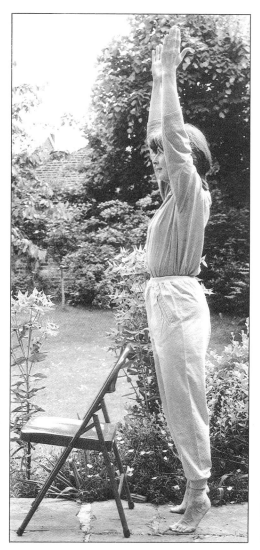

Balancing on one leg

This exercise helps your balance while stretching the front of the lifted thigh and working the muscles of the supporting leg strongly.

Exercise Lift one leg up behind you. Tuck in your buttocks and keep your back straight. Hold the position for thirty seconds, or longer if you can manage it. Repeat with the other leg.

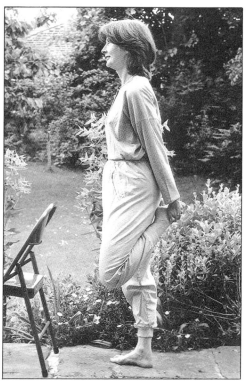

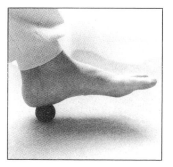

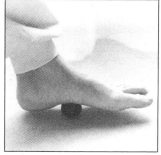

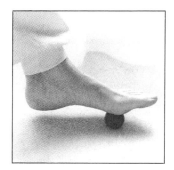

THE PELVIC FLOOR

The pelvic floor muscles

The pelvic floor muscles are like a hammock slung under the pelvis, supporting the abdominal organs, and they need to be strong to resist the pull of gravity. There are three openings in the pelvic floor: the urethra from the bladder, the vagina from the uterus, and the rectum from the bowel. The pelvic floor muscles play an important part in the proper functioning of all these openings. During childbirth the pelvic floor is greatly stretched and it is important to restore its elasticity and strength as quickly as possible after birth.

As we grow older strong muscles in this area continue to be important to avoid the embarrassing problem of incontinence, or, more seriously, to avoid prolapse – collapsing of the vaginal walls (see p.26). Exercising the pelvic floor muscles is a habit we should all get into. Keeping them healthy will increase the circulation to the area and can help to prevent dryness of the vaginal walls often experienced at this age (see p.18).

Checking the strength of your pelvic floor

This area of your body can suffer from lack of exercise in the same way as any other, but if you have neglected to work these muscles it is never too late to start. To check the strength of your pelvic floor try this test. When you next pass urine, try to stop the flow completely in mid-stream, re-start and then stop again. Alternatively, when you make love, squeeze your partner's penis with your pelvic floor muscles. He should be able to feel the muscles tightening. Love-making will become even more pleasurable for both partners if your muscles are strong.

After a tiring day or a long car journey, doing the following exercises in combination with correcting your posture will invigorate you and relieve any heaviness or drag in the lower back and

The pelvic floor muscles

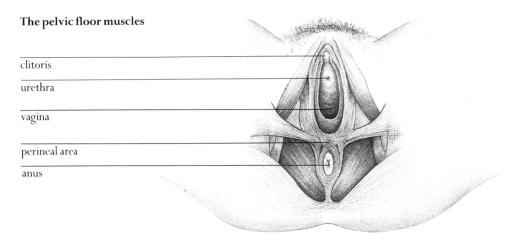

clitoris

urethra

vagina

perineal area

anus

pelvic region. Try to get into the habit of tightening the pelvic floor as often as possible throughout the day – when you are waiting at traffic lights, or in the queue at the supermarket, while answering the telephone or doing the cooking – you should be able to practise the exercises while sitting, standing, lying down or moving around.

Pelvic floor lifts

This exercise should be performed several times daily. Some experts say you should do at least fifty pelvic floor lifts a day, but certainly three or four lifts four times a day is a minimum. You may find this difficult to begin with, but try to increase the number of contractions progressively until you are doing them frequently throughout the day.

The best way to start exercising your pelvic floor is while lying down, since you are not working against gravity. Later on you should practise them in other positions. You can do these exercises anywhere, and no-one will ever know!

Exercise Lie comfortably on the floor with a cushion under your head, knees bent, feet flat and hip-width apart, arms by your sides.

Start with long slow 'lifts', tightening the muscles around your anus, vagina and front passage in one smooth contraction. Imagine you are going up in a lift, squeezing and pulling up the muscles a little tighter each time, as you stop at each 'floor'. See how many 'floors' you can manage – aim to reach the fourth at least!

Hold the last squeeze for a moment as you breathe normally and then gradually release, floor by floor.

Make sure that you are not holding your breath or creating tension elsewhere in the body – concentrate on the movement of the pelvic floor, and relax the rest of your body in the way described on p.119.

Always finish with a squeeze back up to the first floor to keep the muscles contracted.

Progression When you have finished the slow contractions of the muscles, try doing some short, firm squeezes – rather like clenching and letting go of your fist.

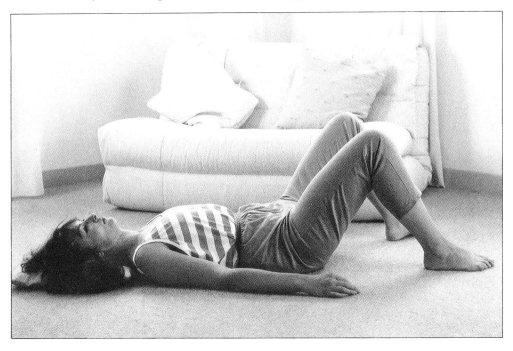

LEARNING TO RELAX

Relaxation and stress

The ability to relax is an important ingredient for a healthy, fulfilled life. Indeed, it is essential if we are to cope with the stresses and irritations of the modern world. We all have to tolerate some forms of stress at one time or another; work, growing children, ageing parents, financial worries, marital differences, ill health – the situations are endless.

What is stress?

But 'stress' is a word that is greatly misused. For a start, it is not always bad. Everyone needs some *positive* stress in their lives – it stimulates action and lends the drive, energy and ambition to attack everyday and long-term problems. For instance, you may have been putting off doing some essential household repairs. Now, perhaps, you have decided to sell the house as the children have left home; you suddenly find the energy to do what is necessary to bring your house up to scratch before putting it on the market. It is a stressful situation, but its effect on you is beneficial.

Stress becomes *negative* – and therefore harmful – when challenges are unable to be met, resulting in fatigue, discouragement, anxiety and depression because of the inability to cope. This situation can lead to a state of *distress*, resulting in sleeplessness, exhaustion, even breakdown (see p. 60).

Recognizing stress

There are many symptoms which may indicate stress, but they are so often ignored. Some people tend to be caught up in a spiral of activity, precisely because they wish to hide their true feelings from themselves, while others become slow and lethargic. No two people react to stress in quite the same way, so it is important to become aware of what affects you personally and to recognize your own anxieties and reactions to stressful situations.

How relaxation can help

In both positive and negative states of stress, relaxation can help. In the former, it gives you a chance to rest and restore your energy. When suffering from over-stress, or distress, learning to relax can help you to control yourself, so that you are better able to reassess your problems and approach them in a more positive light. By developing some form of relaxation technique, you can learn to modify your behaviour, preventing tension from building up and allowing stress to work for you rather than against you.

Relaxation and high blood pressure

Stress can affect your health in one particularly direct way. It is a major cause of hypertension (high blood pressure), and it is especially harmful if you are suffering from this condition already (see p. 23). Relaxation is one of the best preventions of and treatments for high blood pressure, and you should try to relax in the way described below as often as possible if hypertension is likely to be a problem for you. Learning how to relax in any situation, however stressful, is a very worthwhile achievement.

A technique for relaxation

There are as many ways to relax as there are people. It is a very individual thing. A number of methods of relaxation have been developed, some concentrating on relaxing the body and others, more meditative, concentrating on the mind. The Mitchell Method given here is based on the one devised by Laura Mitchell (see Bibliography, p. 124), and is a simple, physiological way of dealing with stress in many different situations.

The ideal time to practise relaxation is after exercise, when the body is warm, and the muscles and joints stretched and mobile. However, once you have mastered the technique, try to incorporate it into your everyday life. It should take you only a few minutes to induce the physiological effects of relaxation.

Body position Lie on your back on a flat, firm surface and cover yourself with a blanket to maintain the warmth of the body. (You will not be able to relax if you are cold.) If your lower back feels uncomfortable, place a cushion under your thighs. Use one under your head also if you wish.

Head and shoulders Press the back of your head gently into the support, pull your shoulders down and lengthen the back of the neck. Then release.

Arms and hands Push your elbows away from your body and place your hands on your abdomen. Stretch your fingers apart and release.

Back and pelvis Push the length of your spine down into the floor and do a small pelvic tilt. Release. Your head and body should feel heavy and relaxed.

Legs and feet Flex your feet away from you, and stretch your legs. Wriggle your toes. Release, allowing your legs to roll out from the hips.

Eyes, face and mouth Close your lids softly over your eyes. Draw the lower jaw down so that the top and bottom teeth no longer touch. The lips should be softly closed, the tongue resting in the bottom of the mouth. Allow the brow, cheeks and jaw to be smooth, slack and relaxed.

Breathing Take a good deep breath and sigh the air slowly out. As you become more relaxed your breathing will become softer. You should gradually be aware of a stillness and calm in your body as you relax; try to allow these feelings to be echoed in your mind.

When you have finished relaxing have a good stretch, roll over on to your side and sit up slowly, as shown on page 74.

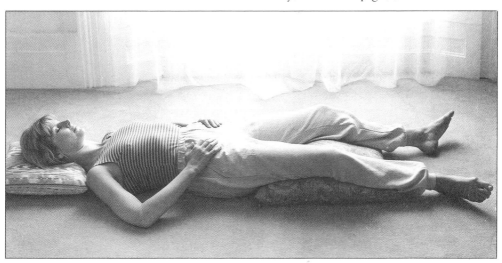

DAILY PROGRAMME

This section, and the Weekly Programme given opposite, will help you see at a glance which exercises you should do every day, and how often, and those which can be done less frequently. Try to do the following at least once a day; asterisks mark the most important. NB If you are unwell or are suffering from back pain or painful arthritis, check with your doctor before proceeding with the Exercise Programme.

BASIC SKILLS: POSTURE

*Correct sitting p.68

*Correct standing p.70

Practise whenever you think about it.

BREATHING

*Check your breathing p.72
3 or 4 deep breaths.

THE FACE

Neck firmer p.76

Facial squeeze and stretch p.76

Chin wag p.77

8 times each after brushing your teeth at night.

NECK AND SHOULDERS

*Head rolling and turning p.78

Shoulder lift p.79

Shoulder circling p.80

8 times each.

ARMS AND HANDS

Underarm stretch and wrist mobilizer p.84
8 times each.

Finger flexing and stretching p.84
8 times each.

THE ABDOMINAL MUSCLES

Side bends p.92
Hold each position for at least 20 seconds.

THE BACK

*Back strengthener and ham-string stretch p.104

Back strengthener and inside thigh stretch p.105

Alternate these exercises and their progressions to your own strength, each day, for 2 minutes.

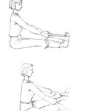

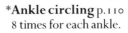

LEGS AND FEET

*Calf strengthener progression p.113
Do the more strenuous progression of this exercise for as long as it takes to become breathless. Alternatively take some other form of strenuous exercise e.g. running for the bus, climbing the stairs.

*Ankle circling p.110
8 times for each ankle.

Arch strengtheners p.111
4 times for each foot.

Toe stretch p.111
4 times for each foot.

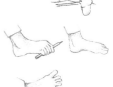

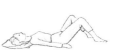

THE PELVIC FLOOR

*Pelvic floor lifts p.117
At least 10 slow and 10 quick lifts as often as possible during the day.

RELAXATION

*A technique for relaxation p.119
5 to 10 minutes every day.

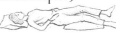

WEEKLY PROGRAMME

If you cannot manage all the exercises in this section every day, to start with concentrate on the ones given opposite in the Daily Programme. Three times a week, set aside more time to include those given below. As you become stronger you may well find that you will want to do both programmes every day, perhaps morning and evening.

ARMS AND HANDS

Full arm stretch p.83
8 times.

Arm and shoulder strengthener p.85
8 times.

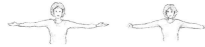

THE ABDOMINAL MUSCLES

Waist twists p.93
Hold each position for at least 20 seconds.
(NB Do not attempt this exercise if you have a history of back pain.)

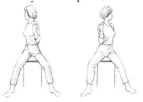

Curl down p.97
Curling up p.100
Alternate these exercises on different days, 8 times each.

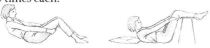

Spine stretch p.99
To follow Curl Down or Curling Up, above.

Diagonal twists p.96
1 to 2 minutes. Try to set up a comfortable rhythm.

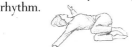

BUTTOCKS AND THIGHS

Outside thigh strengthener p.106
8 times with each leg.

Buttock squeeze with pelvic tilt p.108
8 times.

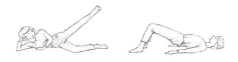

LEGS AND FEET

Knee bends p.109
8 times with each leg.

Calf strengthener p.112
Up and down until the calf aches.

Calf stretch p.113
Hold for at least 20 seconds.

Improving your balance p.114
Balance for 30 seconds or more.

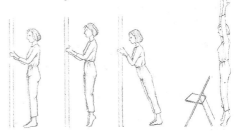

MASSAGE

Self-massage p.82
Do this whenever your neck and shoulders feel tense.

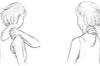

Foot massage p.114
Do this whenever your feet ache.

SPORT & THE OLDER WOMAN

With your new-found fitness you may decide to take up some new activity or sport, but do choose one which suits your ability and life-style and one which you will enjoy. When deciding on a suitable sport, probably the most important factor to be taken into consideration is time. It is essential to choose an activity which fits into your busy schedule, so that you can have time to warm up properly beforehand and cool down afterwards to avoid any injury or stiffness. Try to choose one which you can do throughout the year and which is easily accessible. Do not try to do something too strenuous before you are fit enough to cope

with it or you will become quickly discouraged and give up. If you have had a long break from exercise due to illness or some other reason, work up to your previous fitness level gradually to avoid strain and injury.

There are so many different activities to choose from. Some of the most common are listed here in alphabetical order, together with their relative merits and a few warnings. The sport or leisure activity that you decide upon may not be included, but you will be able to assess its suitability for you by comparing it to a similar one mentioned below.

Cycling

This is ideal, being available to everyone, practical and energy saving. It is excellent for stamina, and can increase the fitness of the heart and lungs and strengthen muscles. Invest in a large bicycle basket or good paniers and start going shopping on your bicycle. Join friends at weekends and explore new areas of your neighbourhood. The possibilities are endless. Do make sure the bicycle is the correct wheel size for you and that handlebars and saddle are adjusted to your height, so that you can work on your posture, keeping your back straight and your shoulders down. Avoid drop handlebars as they force you into a more uncomfortable position in the interests of speed which is not good for the back and neck.

Dancing

A year-round and very social activity, which is also fun. There are numerous clubs providing classes in many different types of dancing, which can be very energetic, or slow, graceful and relaxing. It is a good all-round body conditioning activity. Be careful of so-called 'aerobic dance' classes; if they are not run by reputable, trained instructors you may lay yourself open to strain or even injury.

Golf

This is a less energetic sport than some others, but has the advantage of being quite widely available, social and healthy as you are out in the air and walking fairly long distances. It is particularly good for co-ordination and balance and is a relaxing activity. However it can be quite expensive to join a popular private club.

Horse-riding

Riding through pleasant countryside is a very relaxing pastime. It is also good for muscle strength and co-ordination and a good year-round sport in the fresh air, but beware of falls if you suffer from osteoporosis (see p. 20). Again, it is fairly expensive to do on a regular basis, whether you own your own horse or not.

Jogging and running

These two sports have become very popular over the last few years but beware! Many people have tried to jog or run too far and too fast, not taking into account their level of fitness, and injuries and strain have resulted from this. However, these sports do appear to stimulate the release of natural chemicals in the blood which make the runner feel good.

You should build up your distance and time gradually, becoming aware of your body's reactions, and taking particular care of your knee and ankle joints. Be careful not to jar your spine when you run, by using the whole of the sole of the foot, landing through the heel and springing off from the balls of the feet. If you feel any pain do not attempt to run again until you are free from any discomfort. When performed carefully and gradually, jogging and running are excellent ways of getting and keeping fit, being good for the heart and lungs, increasing muscle strength and endurance, producing a nice 'tiredness' at the end of the session. They have the added advantage of being accessible to anyone, at any time of the year: you can run anywhere. However, do invest in a good pair of running shoes, and avoid running in fog or 'smog'.

Sailing

A good outdoor activity which can be as demanding as you choose to make it! It is good for muscle stamina. A relaxing and social sport, it also can be expensive, although investing in a small sailing dinghy and trailer does mean you can sail regularly even in quite restricted waters.

Ski-ing (down-hill)

This is not something to start in late middle age since the danger to brittle bones from falls is great (see p. 20). However it is an excellent and very invigorating sport – good for muscle strength and endurance, flexibility, particularly of the knees and feet, and good for balance and co-ordination. Unfortunately it is expensive and not always easily accessible.

Ski-ing (cross-country)

Many older people choose to try cross-country ski-ing rather than the faster down-hill kind. It has all the same advantages, but without the same danger of falls, but again access can be difficult.

Skipping

An activity which can be performed anywhere.

It is good for muscle stamina and for the heart and lungs, but again be careful of joint strain and any jarring of the spine.

Squash

A lot of people take up squash because it is easily available, can be over in half an hour or so and is thus suitable for people with busy lives. However the sport has had some adverse publicity recently because it is not one to be performed by the unfit. All too often not enough care is taken to warm up first with a few stretching exercises, and people tend to play a hard, fast game too soon, which can lead to muscle damage. Worse still, strain can be put on the heart, so avoid this sport unless you are already fit.

Do not try to *get* fit playing squash – it is only for *keeping* fit.

Swimming

Swimming is probably the best all-round sport there is. It uses the heart and lungs efficiently, increases muscle strength and stamina, and improves the flexibility of the joints. It is relaxing and easily available. It is also very useful if you are recovering from an injury, or suffer from arthritis, bronchitis, migraine or obesity.

Tennis

Tennis is another sport which can be played at various levels. It can be fast and competitive, or slower and fun. It does tend to concentrate on specific muscle groups, namely the arm you play with and the legs, but the more energetically you play the more muscles you will be using and the more it will improve the performance of your heart and lungs. It is a good social sport and usually fairly easily available: a 'doubles' game is an ideal activity for older couples.

Walking

This is another good all-round activity, available to everyone. A brisk walk uses the heart and lungs efficiently and increases stamina. It is good for co-ordination and produces a pleasant relaxed feeling when you get home!

BIBLIOGRAPHY

Alive and Well and Over 40 Kay Sullivan, 1984
Disorders of Sexual Desire
    Helen Singer Kaplan, 1979
Enjoy Sex in the Middle Years
    Dr Christine E. Sandford, 1983
Exercise for the Over 50s Dr Russell Gibbs, 1981
Everywoman's Life-Guide
    Dr Miriam Stoppard, 1982
50-Plus Life-Guide Dr Miriam Stoppard, 1983
The Health and Fitness Handbook
    Edited by Miriam Polunin, 1981
Human Sexual Inadequacy
    W. H. Masters and V. E. Johnson, 1966
Liberating Masturbation Betty Dodson, 1979
Living Through Middle Age
    Edited by Edith Rudinger, 1976
Menopause – A Positive Approach
    Rosetta Reitz, 1977
My Secret Garden Nancy Friday, 1975
The New Sex Therapy Helen Singer Kaplan, 1978
No More Hot Flashes Penny Wise Rudoff, 1983

Our Bodies Ourselves
    Boston Women's Health Collective, 1978
Principles of Anatomy and Physiology
    Tortora and Anagnostakos, 1984
The Relaxation Response
    Herbert Benson, MD, 1977
Report on Female Sexuality Shere Hite, 1981
Report on Male Sexuality Shere Hite, 1978
Simple Movement
    Laura Mitchell and Barbara Dale, 1980
Simple Relaxation Laura Mitchell, 1977
Soft Exercise – The Complete Book of Stretching
    Arthur Balaskas and John Stirk, 1983
The Stress Factor Donald Norfolk, 1979
Stress and Relaxation Jane Madders, 1978
Unfinished Business Maggie Scarf, 1980
Woman-care
    American Medical Association, 1981
Woman's Experience of Sex Sheila Kitzinger, 1983
Women Coming of Age Jane Fonda, 1984

USEFUL ADDRESSES

Fitness

The Sports Council,
    16 Upper Woburn Place, London, WC1H 0QP.
    01-388 1277
Australia Australian Council for Health,
    Physical Education and Recreation,
    PO Box 1, Kingswood,
    South Australia 5062.
South Africa South African Sports Federation,
    PO Box 1481, Pretoria 0001, South Africa.
Womens League of Health and Beauty,
    18 Charing Cross Road, London, WC2.
    01-240 8456
Auckland, New Zealand Mrs Nina North,
    Mill Road, RD, Bombay, SA.
    Mrs Kay Rhodes, 33 Onslow Road,
    Mount Albert, SA.
South Africa Miss B. Keys,
    13 Killarney Court, Protea Road,
    Newlands, Cape.

General Health

Women's National Cancer Control Campaign,
    1 South Audley Street, London, W1Y 5DQ.
    01-499 7532
Mastectomy Association (in Association
    with National Society for Cancer Relief),
    26 Harrison Street, off Gray's Inn Road,
    King's Cross, London, WC1H 8JG.
    01-837 0908
Australia Australian Cancer Society Inc.,
    PO Box 135, Civic Square, ACT 2608.
    (062) 480 726
South Africa The National Cancer Association,
    Northern Transvaal Branch, PO Box 275,
    Pretoria 0001, RSA.
Menopause Clinics – contact your local
    Health Authority.
Women's Health Concern,
    17 Earls Terrace, London, W8. 01-602 6669
    (For menopause counselling.)

Alcoholics Anonymous,
  11 Redcliffe Gardens, London, SW10.
  01-352 9779 (See also your local telephone
  directory.)
Australia General Service Office,
  363 George Street, Room 301, 3rd floor,
  GPO Box 5321,
  Sydney, NSW, Aus. 2001.
South Africa General Service Office,
  504 Delbree House, 300 Bree Street,
  PO Box 23005, Joubert Park, 2044, SA.

ASH (Action on Smoking and Health),
  5/11 Mortimer Street, London, W1.

The Migraine Trust,
  45 Great Ormond Street, London, WC1.
  01-278 2676

Family Planning Association,
  27 Mortimer Street, London, W1.
  01-636 7866
Australia Australian Federation of Family
  Planning Associations,
  70 George Street, Sydney,
  New South Wales 2000.
New Zealand New Zealand Family Planning
  Association,
  PO Box 68200, Newton Auckland 1.
South Africa Family Planning Association
  of South Africa,
  412 York House, 46 Kerk Street,
  Johannesburg 2001.

Back Pain Association,
  31-33 Park Road, Teddington,
  Middlesex, TW11 0AB. 01-977 5474

Arthritis Care,
  6 Grosvenor Crescent, London, SW1.
  (Welfare and rehabilitation centre, branches
  nationwide.) 01-235 0902
Australia Arthritis Foundation of Australia,
  12th floor, Wynyard House,
  291 George Street, Sydney, NSW 2000.
New Zealand Arthritis and Rheumatism
  Foundation of New Zealand,
  PO Box 10-020, Southern Cross Building,
  Brandon Street, Wellington, NZ.

Marriage, Family and Relationships

National Marriage Guidance Council,
  Herbert Gray College,

Little Church Street, Rugby, CV21 3AP.
  (See also your local telephone directory.)
Australia National Marriage Guidance Council
  of Australia,
  6 Morton Road, Burwood, Victoria, 3125.
South Africa Cape Town Marriage Guidance
  Council,
  309 Groote Kirk Building, Cape Town.
New Zealand National Marriage Guidance
  Coucil of New Zealand,
  PO Box 2728, Wellington.

Institute of Family Therapy,
  43 New Cavendish Street, London, W1.
  01-935 1657

CRUSE (National Organisation for the
  Widowed and their Children),
  126 Sheen Road, Richmond,
  Surrey, PW9 1UR. 01-940 4818

Association of Sex and Marital Therapists,
  The Whiteley Wood Clinic,
  Woofindin Road, Sheffield S10 3TL.

Divorce Conciliation and Advisory Service,
  38 Ebury Street, London SW1. 01-730 2422
Australia Marriage Divorce Counselling
  Centre,
  1 Ord Street, Perth 6000.
Marriage, Reconciliation and Separation
  Counselling,
  262 Pitt Street, Sydney, NSW 2000.

The National Council for Carers and their
  Elderly Dependents Ltd,
  29 Chilworth Street, London, W2.
  01-262 1451

Careers

National Advisory Centre on Careers for
  Women,
  Drayton House, 30 Gordon Street,
  London, WC1. 01-380 0117
Over 40s Association for Women Workers,
  120 Cromwell Road, London, SW7.
  01-370 2556
New Directions for Women,
  39 Queen's Road, Richmond upon Thames,
  Surrey.
The Career Development For Women,
  97 Mallard Place, Twickenham,
  Middlesex, TW1 4SW. 01-892 3806

INDEX

ACKNOWLEDGEMENTS

The publishers would like to thank
Dr Sue Morrison and Tony Lycholat
for their help in the preparation of this book.
We would also like to thank the following people
for allowing us to photograph them:
Esther Caplin; Steve and Wendy Corduner; Eve de Meza and Benjamin;
Kiffy Driscoll; Freddie and Naomi Earlle; Claude Harz;
Sophie Hastings; Rosie Keegan, Cassy, Carly and Bella;
Rita Kelleher; Lysie Kihl; Marian Kihl; Jane Lagesse;
John and Wendy Morgan; Dulcie Morrell; Helge Rubinstein;
Pippa Rubinstein and Jolyon; Anthea Sieveking; Nena Thorley.
Thanks are also due to BUPA Medical Centre
for providing reference for illustration.

Illustrations by Elaine Anderson

Photograph on p. 7 by Alan Stewart

Editor Nicky Adamson
Art Editor Caroline Hillier

Series Editor Pippa Rubinstein
Art Director Debbie MacKinnon

Filmset by SX Composing Ltd, Rayleigh, Essex
Origination by F. E. Burman Ltd, London
Printed and bound in Yugoslavia

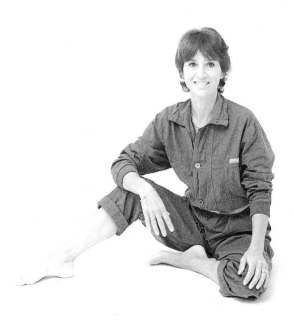